Pelican Books

Dec. 1971.

Love, Sex and Being Human

Paul Bohannan was born in the Middle Western
heartland of the United States, and grew up in a
rather peripatetic manner throughout its western
half. His education includes a B.A. from the
University of Arizona in Anthropology and
German Literature, and three degrees from Oxford
which he attended as a Rhodes Scholar. He was a
Lecturer in Social Anthropology at Oxford for
five years, then returned to the United States to
go to Princeton, and finally came to rest at
Northwestern University.

He first went to Africa in 1949, and spent over
two and a half years with the Tiv of Central
Nigeria. He has also done field work in Kenya,
and has travelled widely in the continent. His
books include *Justice and Judgment Among the
Tiv*, *African Homicide and Suicide*, *Tiv Economy*,
Markets in Africa, *Social Anthropology*, *African
Outline* (a Penguin Book) and *Divorce and After*.

Paul Bohannan

Love, Sex and Being Human

A Book about the
Human Condition for
Young People

Penguin Books

Penguin Books Ltd, Harmondsworth,
Middlesex, England
Penguin Books Australia Ltd, Ringwood,
Victoria, Australia

First published in the U.S.A. by Doubleday 1969
Published in Great Britain by Pelican Books 1970
Copyright © Paul Bohannan, 1969

Made and printed in Great Britain by
C. Nicholls & Company Ltd
Set in Monotype Times

The line illustrations for this book
were prepared by the Graphic Arts Division of the
American Museum of Natural History

'No morality is an absolute, the safely proven, the caught bird with salt on its tail. It is the chosen and the hoped-for, a loyalty that is man's burden, his glory, and his cross. For in the last analysis every culture is a moral geometry – a system *not* inalternatively imbedded in the physical world, but a contingent means of triangulating one's course through reality.'

Weston La Barre

Contents

Illustrations/tables

Preface

I am not advocating any specific moral behaviour. I have tried to make this book factual. The facts are taken from biology, anatomy, physiology, medicine (including psychiatry), psychology, sociology, and anthropology.

I am advocating one specific idea: that human behaviour best results from individual and community awareness and decision, reached on the basis of accurate knowledge of alternatives rather than on the basis of fear or superstition. There can be knowledge about ethics and morality as well as about anatomy.

I have some values of my own that sometimes show. Human beings can be aware of and comfortable with their animal natures. They can be taught and loved when they are young so that as adults they can be loving and cultured teachers of the young. They can be helped by parents and teachers, neighbours and doctors to reach autonomy – that magnificent state of individual spontaneous euphoria which makes predictable social relationships a joy, work and recreation a source of pleasure, and things and people a constant reaffirmation of the worth of the self and of the species.

Some of the specialists who have read this book in manuscript have asked whether I really expect teenagers to come to overt decisions about the way in which they will devise their own moralities. The answer is 'Of course – they do already.' None of my teenage readers and critics raised this question. If teenagers cannot do it – cannot inquire about and learn the moral postures and facts of the communities in which they live, cannot make an overt and usable personal morality – then it may well be their informants who are at fault.

Preface

The communications gap between the generations is not really due to age difference or even to cultural difference. It is a matter of role behaviour. The adult role is too often defined to be to give children the norms, not the facts. Children are quick to perceive the credibility gap, and they come to think of parents, teachers, and clergymen as hypocritical. Adults also perceive the gap – and say that the process of becoming adult means to learn for one's self how to compromise with 'reality'. Both are correct.

Thus, to children, adult informants seem to be shot through with faults, and hence their moral standards for compromise seem to be 'lies' and hypocrisy. Unfortunately, they sometimes turn against the adult world, and use the 'lies' as an excuse for amorality or immorality – even by their own standards. The adults wonder, 'What did we do wrong?'

The answer is that standards of truthtelling must be revised. In today's world, both the role of adult (including those of parent, teacher, clergyman) and the role of children and adolescents must be examined. Penicillin and the pill have made imperative new standards of truthtelling about sex.

Acknowledgements

The quotation from Weston La Barre that begins this book is to be found in his *The Human Animal*, University of Chicago Press, 1954, p. 221. The lines from Walt Whitman at the end of the book form the last stanza of 'A Woman Waits for Me' from *Leaves of Grass*, 1860.

I want to thank Nathaniel S. French, the headmaster of the North Shore Country Day School, and that school's parents and teachers' committee for turning my attention to this subject. I want to thank the freshman class of 1965–66 at the school, who were patient and co-operative with my first struggles to communicate with people like them. I sometimes had to simplify my language to explain concepts, but I soon found that I must never simplify the message or they would know that they were being cheated. My gratitude is in response to their magnificent candour.

Literally scores of teenagers, parents, teachers, clergymen, and physicians have helped me with this book. I shall try to send each of them a thank-you copy, but I hope that they will forgive me for not listing them here – I do not want to pretend to the expertness that their names might imply. What is in this book is mine, for all that I have been helped with it (as I have with every other aspect of my life) by my family, my friends, my colleagues, and my students.

Paul Bohannan

Part One

The Biological Basis of Sexuality

Chapter 1

The Human Animal

Human beings are animals. They have to deal with everything that implies. Any morality that denies the animal nature of human beings will ultimately collapse.

Human beings are also social creatures. As they adapt their actions to one another, they evaluate those actions in terms of good and bad. Any morality that denies the ethical foundation of human society will also ultimately collapse.

This book is about one of the animal drives – sexuality – and about human evaluation of it. My goal is to be as frank and objective about the morality of sex as about the biology.

In today's world, the facts of biology are acceptable to most people – they are considered to be facts. But morality is put in a different sphere – morality, it would seem, is not considered to be factual. Yet, it is not mere biological fact that people have to know in order to get along. They also have to know something about the good and bad effects of what they do. It is not the physiology of the sexual organs or even techniques of sexual intercourse that make for difficult discussion between the generations. Rather we are hung up on questions of morality. 'Male and female' is a fairly easy subject. 'Good and bad' is a very difficult subject.

Human Beings Are Mammals

Human beings exhibit the classifying characteristics of mammals in what they have (in the flush of rediscovery) come to think of as an exaggerated form. Probably man is no more the arch-mammal than he is the arch-angel. But from the human viewpoint, made poignant by the new insights of science, he certainly seems to be both.

Mammals are warm-blooded animals that reproduce sexually, bear live young in a remarkably immature state, and nurse these young for an extended period of time at the breasts of – and, among human beings and other primates, under the eyes of – the female. Except for marsupials such as kangaroos, among whom the young move from an internal womb to a pouch that might be compared to an external womb, the human being is born at a more immature state of his physical development than any other mammal.

Moreover, the human being is one of the few animals that are sexually active at all seasons. With the exception of some apes, and of some monkeys in captivity, there is a season for sex among all other animals – for man there is no closed season except those that are socially demanded.

All mammals, including man, have to one degree or another 'specialized' in the brain and central nervous system as a means of evolutionary survival. Man has, through development of brain, ability to think abstractly, and a special capacity to learn, moved into an interesting biological position – he has come to depend on his own thought for survival. Changes in man's culture are very much more rapid than changes in biological form, so that with culture man has a very efficient means for learning to survive (and also, of course, to destroy himself).

Given such a situation, the 'present generation' of human beings always finds itself confronting a puzzling 'black box'. Human instincts – whatever we may mean by that – are so arranged that man has to learn everything he will ever know. Yet human learning equipment is necessarily the equipment for questioning. Man learns to question as he learns – to question himself, his own activities, and his own social institutions. All languages have words for examining man's self and society, his personal and social problems – and these words can move him deeply. Man is – and perhaps this is the only claim he can make to uniqueness among the mammals – the only animal capable of creating and realizing his own moral dilemma.

The moral dilemma is simple to state: Each of us is an individual in a society; each of us perceives himself and feels his own needs and wants; at the same time each of us is dependent on receiving from and giving to other people in our world, and these people impose limitations on us. The moral dilemma is being torn between self and society, when their demands are at odds.

Civilized Western men of the past tried to solve this moral dilemma by turning against their bodies and against their animality. They did this by the simple means of equating animality with evil. Then, everything that was not 'animal' was, by this oversimple logic, 'good'. We are today living in a period in which we are discovering that denial of our animal nature (and mortification of the flesh) does not provide an adequate solution to the moral dilemma.

Man's nature makes it impossible for him not to feel hunger, rage, sexual urges, ambition, love of children.

But man also has a 'second nature' – to utilize and gratify and hence to 'control' this primary nature; the second nature causes him to organize into families and communities and to struggle within status systems – to seek love and security. It is impossible for a normal human being not to have knowledge, attitudes, and moralities. His salvation – like his problem – is that he has a drive for knowledge (because his eyes and hands and brain and his culture demand it) and a need for attitudes that are shared with at least some members of the community who are 'his people'.

Man is an intensely social animal. Although many men, once they are adult, need privacy and perhaps some solitude, they must be brought up in the thick of a society. The people of a society are held together by communications, common ideas, and shared things which anthropologists call culture. One of the most important points about cultures is that they give men guidance about how to view their bodies, their animalness, their human natures, their achievements, and their moral dilemmas.

Mankind has not only developed the capacity for confronting a moral dilemma, he has also created the kind of society that

19

gives him its cultural answers to what is right and what is wrong. He must learn these answers. And, as we have seen, his learning apparatus is also his questioning apparatus.

Learning and questioning is the business of all human beings. Therefore, teaching is also the business of all of us. Teaching can be done in two ways. We can teach by precept – say, 'Do this! Don't do that!' We can also teach by example. The learning process is different in the two cases. One is merely learning facts or techniques. The other is learning feelings, as well as facts and techniques. One method is by memorizing. The other is by identifying.

The grave difficulty for man comes when what he learns by memorization is different from what he learns by identification. In the past, sex has been one of the topics about which there has been the greatest of contradictions between what was learned in these two ways. Young people are still admonished to do one thing by people who themselves behave quite differently. In correcting this situation, there is no substitute for accurate facts: facts about what we are, facts about what we say we should do, and facts about what, being human, we actually do.

The Human Dilemma

The situation is, thus, a simple one. Human beings are mammals, and perennially sexed mammals at that – there is no season at which sex can be forgotten. Human beings are social mammals capable of intense love of their young. They are also capable of speech, learning, and ultimately of moral dilemmas. They are capable of lifting the concept of 'love' out of its parent-child relationship, generalizing it, and giving it new moral dimensions. They can even apply it to ideas about the deity, about a moral attitude towards mankind as a whole, and – here is the most amazing fact – they can even use the idea and emotion of love both to control and to enrich mammalian sexuality.

The dilemma is the more puzzling because there is no one 'right' way to do this. Different societies exhibit different moralities; morality changes from one historical period to the next. So it looks, to a person seeking for a way of life, as if he is called upon to determine which actions to take and which to avoid when the alternatives are not clear-cut and when the consequences are not certain. The solution to the dilemma is not to be found in any single 'answer', but rather in an understanding of the process for finding answers. *That* is where we are hung up.

To tackle this dilemma, all of us must learn to be as factual as we can about all parts of man's nature – in doing so all of us are underlining our own nature. I shall start this book with the biology of sex – but, let it be remembered, in today's world the biology is easy. We can be frank about it; most of us can examine our own bodies without humiliation or guilt.

The second part of the book is about social morality. And that part is not so easy. It is not possible for most of us to look at our attitudes as coolly as we can look at our bodies. But that is the task we must set ourselves; we must forge our moral positions from our social and biological natures. This book is an attempt in that direction.

Chapter 2

Men and Women

When a child is born, the first question everyone asks about 'it' is whether 'it' is a boy or a girl. When people know that, they know how to act towards the mother, the father, and towards the child.

From birth to death, a person is assigned to one of the two sexual categories. Either he is male or she is female. Only strangers refer to a baby as a mere baby. Everyone else, particularly the parents and family and the friends of the family, sees the child as a girl or a boy, and acts accordingly.

Growing as Male or Female

The differences in the way people treat males and females, thus, begin to show up early in life. If you go into the maternity ward of a modern hospital, you will find that the nurses lift and handle girl babies differently from boy babies. If you see them only in the starched precision of formal paternal viewings, the differences may not look very great. But if you watch them when they are playing with a baby as much for their own pleasure as for that of the baby, you will see the differences immediately. The nurses pick up girls with smaller gestures. They do not move them as far or as rapidly, and they use higher tones of voice than they do to boy babies. They touch girls more gently. They tend to pick up boy babies with large, sweeping gestures, to speak more loudly to them, and to touch them a little bit more roughly.

Mothers do the same thing. Mothers – especially experienced

mothers – go on the assumption (even if it is not stated) that boys are stronger than girls, and that girls must be better protected. The mothers, like the nurses, react to the baby not just as a baby, but as a son or daughter.

The difference in the way people treat boys and girls increases as the child grows older, so that finally as an adult you are always conscious that the way you treat a man is far different from the way you treat a woman – and that statement is true whether you are a man or a woman.

Because your body is either male or female, and because all of the people you know treat you in the ways they have been taught to think are suitable for either males or females, you obviously develop into a more or less masculine or a more or less feminine person.

Every society assigns different qualities of personality to men and to women; every society expects to find those qualities, and usually does. The people of the society assign jobs and rewards in accordance with what they think are socially appropriate male and female jobs and male and female rewards.

There is probably no quality that is so important or so far-reaching in determining the course of your social life as the fact of your sex. Indeed, European women are in some ways – womanly ways – more like Pygmy women than they are like European men; they share experiences of motherhood and feelings of domestic responsibility and feminine sexuality – far more subtle than the differences in European and Pygmy culture. In just the same way, European men have in common with Chinese men or African men the bond of being responsible, strong, questing males, for all that they share the bond of a common culture with American women.

All these facts – that you are either male or female, that you experience the world as such, and that you are treated as such – are so natural as to seem commonplace. But they are very important. In the process of being male, you are treated as a male by men – and also by women. The way that men treat a small male is very different from the way women treat a small male. In order to be a full-fledged male, you have to learn to deal with

23

both men and women. You learn while you are growing up how to be a male among males or a female among females. That is very different from dealing with the opposite sex, which you must also learn.

In order to be fully himself, each person must react to both men and women. Every person needs models on which to base and gauge his own behaviour – he needs both male and female models. You must, in short, learn something about what you are not as well as what you are.

A great deal has been written about the qualities of males and of females. Every society has ideas about the masculine and the feminine, and holds them to be 'common sense'. In our own society it is said that males are more aggressive than females, and that females are conversely gentler and more easily trained, or, indeed, 'domesticated'. It is certainly true that in our own society, females learn a longer attention span earlier in their lives than do males, and learn to sit still at a younger age. It is said – in the Western world at least – that men are stronger and that females are 'the weaker sex'. This is repeated in spite of the fact that all of the figures collected by insurance companies show that women have a longer life expectancy than men, and that they seem capable of enduring great hardship and strain, and that they are not so delicate physically as men are. The men, we might say, are the strong ones, but the women are the tough ones.

In America, it is even said that women are more intuitive than men, but that men use their brains better. We do not know whether this is a quality of the male or female mind and body because we certainly, in these same societies, teach boys not to follow their intuition but to use their heads, and we withhold equal rewards for the same brainwork from women.

Most of these commonsense sayings are tales which have been neither proved nor disproved by science. So long as you ask the question whether men or women are 'better', you will never find an answer. Men and women are not comparable on the basis of good and bad, but only on the basis of how well they perform the tasks that their bodies and their societies set for them.

It is, of course, true that as adults women must bear the children, and their lives must be geared, to at least some degree, to menstruation and childbearing. This tends to put women in a dependent position on men for at least a few years during their lives. During those years, the horizons of their lives are more circumscribed than are the horizons of their men, who must go out and deal with the outside world. Women in such a situation are obliged to become highly conscious of the emotional tone within the comparatively small family and neighbourhood groups. During the same period of time, men are required to become aware and to use their minds and muscles in a larger social arena, and one that is generally not so highly charged emotionally. Men are, in at least a few of their experiences, thrust aside from the elementary family experiences – the birth and early care of children. A man's importance is in begetting children, loving and caring for the child's mother, and ultimately enjoying being a good example and a good teacher to the children. The importance of a man's role as father grows as the child becomes older and needs a pattern with which he can identify. The woman's importance is in carrying and bearing the child, feeding it, caring for it, and setting a standard for the maternal love that will eventually be given to even the third generation.

In most societies a mother's task is important well into the physical adulthood of her child. But it is nevertheless (particularly if it is well done) a task of diminishing scope as the child grows older and hopefully, more independent. A mother must learn to 'let go'. As one sensitive psychologist has put it, she must learn to love her child into independence, and she must have the security herself that will give her pleasure in seeing the child independent.

A father's job follows a different rhythm. He must begin by giving his love and assistance to the baby's mother – and perhaps to the baby too, but so long as he is not hostile to the baby, it is not so important for a year or so as what he does for the mother. Then, as the child begins to learn ideas instead of just raw feelings (which, of course, he has been learning all along), the father comes into his own. Yet, like the mother, he must also learn to

25

'let go'. He too has to trust his child, boy or girl, into independence.

This means that a man must adjust to not being central to all situations of family life; his task is to be the contact of the family with the greater world. Women must adjust to a state of relative social deprivation. During the infancy of their children women may be deprived for a few years of at least some of the wide-ranging experiences that being male allows. Both must also adjust to another kind of deprivation – they must release their children as the child's need for them changes and ultimately diminishes.

In today's world, male and female roles are changing and have changed. More and more women are working. Many are helping to support the family – and some are doing it alone. Men are learning that merely being the only bread-winner does not prove their masculinity; working itself need not make women less feminine. Many women do have the kind of contact with the outer world that used to be characteristic only of men. And, at the same time, many men take on more responsibility for children and get more of their rewards directly within the family. This fact does not prove that women have emasculated their men. It merely proves that the demands on men and women, and the resulting kinds of experience to which each must adjust, are changing as the technology and organization of society changes.

Thus, each of us has the psychic experience of being male or female beginning at birth, and the differences widen as one grows older. Indeed, you will grow old and die either as a male or a female. You may, at several times in your life, wonder what it is like to be the other. And you may even get some gleam of understanding – but it will always be a vicarious understanding. You will never 'know' how the other half lives.

The Need of Men and Women for One Another

If the differences between men and women become greater as they grow up, then the dependency between them increases at the same time. Throughout life men and women need one another as they become more and more differentiated in their experience of the world.

Three different things must be remembered in discussing sex identification.

First, there are bodily differences between males and females. On the basis of physical characteristics, one is given what psychiatrists sometimes call a 'sex of assignment'. You are socially declared to be male or female.

Second, there are psychic differences because of these physiological differences themselves, because of the chemical differences in hormonal balance, and because of the different sense experience that physical and cultural capabilities allow us. Thus, the way we treat other people reacting to our maleness or our femaleness is important in creating in us qualities that will be interpreted as masculine or feminine.

Third, society allows the two sexes different rewards and assigns them different tasks and different modes of behaviour. Every society has a view of how men should behave and how women should behave; the two are always thought to be poles apart in the way in which personalities are judged. Anthropologists, standing back from any specific culture, know that many characteristics that are considered feminine in one society may be considered masculine in another society.

So a male is a creature with a male body, a masculine personality which comes from experiencing the world with his male body and from the lessons he is taught because he is male; he is also, then, someone occupying a man's place in society (however that may be defined in his community). A female is a human creature with a female body, a feminine personality, and a woman's place in society.

Confusing physical, social, and psychic characteristics has led to a lot of unnecessary heartache. 'Sissies' are not homosexuals; driving and efficient women are not 'masculinized' monsters. They are playing certain social roles that allow them to adjust at least some of their psychic needs to the vicissitudes of our social definitions of masculine and feminine. When we judge them, we all too often confuse the criteria of physical sex with the culturally defined notions of masculinity and femininity. Probably there has been more foolishness written on the relationship between a male body and culturally 'masculine' behaviour than on any other single topic in the whole realm of behaviour, unless it be the relationship between a female body and 'feminine' behaviour.

Intuitive understanding is not a female trick – it is a quality that is socially assigned to females; some of them develop it and some do not. Leadership drive and inventiveness, business ability and a good head for figures are not traits that derive from a male body, but rather they are social assignments of the masculine role. Hence, when they are found in males they are rewarded and fostered, as they often are not when found in females.

Chapter 3

Females

Human beings exhibit a rare and interesting form of what biologists call 'sexual dimorphism', which means that males and females have widely differing physical characteristics.

Obviously, sexual dimorphism is a relative matter because even in those species which show it least the sexes are distinguished by the sexual organs. Yet in certain species of birds such as crows it is necessary to dissect the animal to determine its sex, and in some mammals (some field mice and shrews) the sex organs so deteriorate when the mating season is over that scientists cannot tell the difference even with dissection.

The chief distinctiveness of human sexual dimorphism is that both adult males and adult females show exaggerations or differences from characteristics that are shared by both sexes in infancy. In most other species, it is only one sex of the adult animals that shows such specialized non-infantile development. Among gorillas, for example, the male develops many special features while the female differs from infants in little more than size. The human kind of dimorphism, with considerable changes for both sexes, is not a common sort.

Thus not only do men and women differ physically from one another; both differ widely from infants. Men and women differ in their primary sex characteristics or genital organs, and in their secondary sex characteristics – such as the breasts of women and the greater body hair and lower voices for men, and differences in the proportion of the bones (especially in the pelvic region) and in distribution of body fat.

This chapter describes the adult female body, with special

attention to the anatomy of the primary sex characteristics and to the biochemical cycle of ovulation and menstruation. The next chapter deals with the male.

The Female Body

The female skeleton is generally more delicate than the male skeleton, but the two are enough alike that all a scientist can do, when he examines a skeleton, is to assign a probability that it is male or female. Generally, the female pelvis is larger in proportion to the rest of the body; it is more suited to supporting the weight of an unborn child and to the movements of the bones necessitated by the processes of birth. Most men, but not all, have hips narrower than their shoulders; most women, but not all, have hips either slightly broader or about the same as their chests and shoulders.

In the past it was assumed that the legs of the female are also shorter in proportion to total height than those of the male. Again, this fact is true for the average, but there is great overlap and the matter may well be affected by diet and types of exercise in childhood.

Female masculature is not so rugged as that of the male. Although it is possible for women to develop the mighty biceps and other muscles that men may develop, especially if they do the same work and do it as constantly, in most societies the work of women is spread out over more time but is less strenuous at specific times. Thus the muscles in women's bodies seldom develop either the size or the hardness of the muscles in men's bodies.

Female body proportions have changed considerably in the last sixty years. Women are taller and heavier than they were at the turn of the century. Sitting height, girth of chest, girth of waist, and breadth of shoulders have all increased in women since that time. However, the hips have not increased in either breadth or girth. Although we do not know all the precise reasons, female figures are somewhat different today from what they were in grandmother's time.

At the time of puberty, the hormone balance becomes very different in the female body from that of the male. All sex hormones are present in both men and women; however, the amounts and their balance are quite different. It is the changes in hormonal balance at puberty that bring about the development of both the primary and the secondary sex characteristics. The hormones released by the female body as it approaches maturity cause the breasts to develop and the figure to fill out, just as those in the male body lead to the masculine voice and the growth of body hair and beard.

The Primary Sex Characteristics of Females

The main components of the female genitalia are the ovaries, the Fallopian tubes, the uterus or womb, and the vagina, all shown in the accompanying illustrations.

The ovaries. Until recently, scientists believed that at the time of birth, a female body contained as many as 40,000 eggs that might develop to become fertilizable, and that it could never produce more. Within the last few years, however, this view has been challenged by the discovery that apparently eggs can be manufactured in the ovaries during the adult life of a woman. There is no absolute agreement on this matter.

The ovaries are approximately spherical organs, about an inch in length, and weigh about three grammes. Every woman has two deep in her body, one on each side of the uterus. In the sexual cycle of the female, an egg ripens and is released in every period of about four weeks, from one or the other ovary. (It is not certain that the ovaries alternate in production.) On a few occasions, more than one egg will be released from one ovary, or one will be released from each ovary. If both such eggs are fertilized, fraternal twins will be born (identical twins result from division of a single egg and a single sperm, whereas fraternal twins come from two eggs, each of which has been fertilized by a different sperm). The process of releasing an egg is called ovulation; it will be described further in the next section of this chapter.

31

Figure 1. The Female Reproductive System

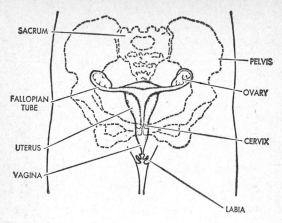

A. The placement of the female reproductive organs within the pelvic girdle.

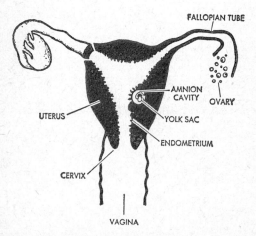

B. The ripened egg is released from the ovary and travels through the Fallopian tube. If it is fertilized, it will, when it reaches the uterus, imbed itself in the endometrium of the uterine wall. If it is not fertilized, it will deteriorate and pass unnoticed out of the body through the vagina.

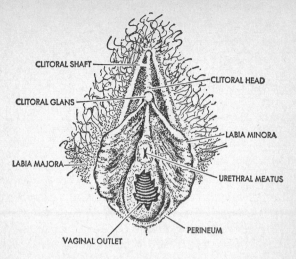

CLITORAL SHAFT

CLITORAL HEAD

CLITORAL GLANS

LABIA MINORA

LABIA MAJORA

URETHRAL MEATUS

PERINEUM

VAGINAL OUTLET

C. The external genitalia.

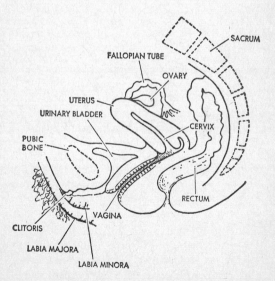

SACRUM

FALLOPIAN TUBE

OVARY

UTERUS

URINARY BLADDER

CERVIX

PUBIC BONE

RECTUM

CLITORIS

VAGINA

LABIA MAJORA

LABIA MINORA

D. A side view of the female reproductive system.

Fallopian tubes. Extending from each ovary, a small tube runs to the upper side of the uterus. The eggs pass through these tubes after leaving the ovaries. The tubes are very tiny – no more than the thickness of a hair at the place where they enter the uterus; they are about four inches long. The egg requires three or four days for passage down the Fallopian tubes. However, it can stay alive for only about a day or a day and a half. If it is not fertilized it disintegrates before it reaches the uterus. If it is fertilized, it descends into the uterus and is imbedded in the inner lining.

The uterus. This organ, also called the womb, is a pear-shaped organ, about three inches long. Its walls are made up of a middle layer of muscle – some of the strongest muscles in the female body. There is an outer layer of membrane, and an inner one of mucous material. The uterus usually is tilted forward, with its mouth, called the cervix, towards the back. The uterus can expand during pregnancy to many times its size. If the egg is fertilized, it attaches itself to the mucous lining of the walls of the uterus and the development of the child begins.

The vagina. The vagina is usually described as a tube or barrel which connects the cervix of the uterus with the external surface of the woman's body. It is about three inches long, but capable of very considerable extension in length. During sexual intercourse the cervix rises, and the vagina lengthens towards the back; this process will be described further in Chapter 5. The function of the vagina is to contain the penis of the sexual partner, and to provide a 'pool' for the seminal fluid of the male in such a position as to allow the cervix to submerge itself in the seminal fluid, which can then flow into the uterus and the Fallopian tubes.

The vulva. The external genitals of the female are called the vulva. They are composed primarily of the clitoris, the opening of the vagina, and the two flaps of flesh called the *labia minora* (small lips) on the inside, and the *labia majora* (large lips) on the outside.

34

The clitoris, as is evident in the accompanying diagram, is a small button-like protrusion at the very top of the vulva. It is homologous to the penis of the male in that it is extremely sensitive, it enlarges in size with excitation, and is covered with a fold of skin like the foreskin (called prepuce in technical language). The clitoris is vital to the sexual excitation and pleasure of the female, but otherwise does not play a functional part in reproduction. Some cultures in the Middle East and Africa (and a few other places) remove it in an operation analogous to male circumcision.

Between the vaginal opening and the clitoris is the urethral meatus – the orifice at which the urethra running from the urinary bladder leaves the body.

In some girls who have never had sexual intercourse, there is a membrane that covers a part of the vaginal outlet. It is called the hymen in technical language, and was known in Middle English as the maidenhead. If the hymen is present – and it may not be – it must be broken before full sexual intercourse can take place. The breaking of the hymen – called 'defloration' – usually occurs in the course of first sexual intercourse, but may have occurred before that time as a result of violent exercise or the misuse of a tampon during menstruation (tampons do not normally cause defloration). The absence of a hymen does not mean that a girl is not a virgin, although its presence usually does mean that she is – there are a few exceptions.

The Menstrual Cycle

The most dramatic aspect of female sexual physiology is the cycle of menstruation and ovulation, which takes place every twenty-eight to thirty days. Like all cycles, it is difficult to know just where to begin in describing it, because – as you can see by reference to the diagram – it is a constantly repeating pattern which goes on all the time from menarche, when it occurs for the first time in a girl's life, until menopause, the 'change of life' during which it ceases.

The cycle is controlled by the pituitary gland, located at the

Figure 2. The Menstrual Cycle

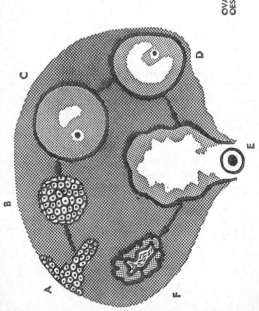

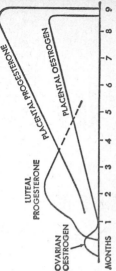

A. The diagrammatic growth of an egg. A and B are newly formed potential egg cells within the ovary; C and D indicate maturation of one of the cells into an egg while surrounding cells develop into a follicle; E shows ovulation while F is the remnants of the follicle, now transformed into a *corpus luteum*.

B. Curves indicating the amounts and the sources of sex hormones present during pregnancy.

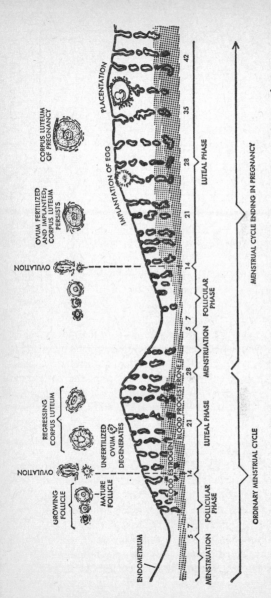

C. Summary of events during menstrual cycle. Top: Ovarian cycle – follicle growth, ovulation, and *corpus luteum* formation. Bottom: Uterine cycle – growth and degeneration of endometrium during ordinary menstrual cycle; growth and maintenance of endometrium during menstrual cycle ending in pregnancy. Variations in concentrations of oestrogen secreted by follicle and progesterone secreted by *corpus luteum* are indicated.

base of the brain. It secretes two hormones which are the prime movers in the cycle. One of these is called F S H (follicle-stimulating hormone) and the other is called L H (luteinizing hormone).

The pituitary secretes F S H, which induces the growth of a follicle in the ovary. The word follicle means 'container' and is applied to several body parts which contain or hold something else – the hair follicle is probably the most widely known. The ovarian follicle contains the human egg. As the follicle matures, it in turn secretes another hormone called oestrogen, which is instrumental in preparing the endometrium, the mucous lining of the uterus, to receive and nourish a fertilized egg. At the same time, oestrogen affects the pituitary so that it begins to secrete L H. When the F S H and the L H reach a particular balance in the body, the mature follicle releases the developed egg into one of the Fallopian tubes.

After the egg has been ejected, the follicle is called the *corpus luteum* – 'yellow body'. Under the stimulation of L H, the *corpus luteum* produces another hormone, progesterone. Progesterone inhibits further ovulation and maintains the endometrium in the uterus. If the egg is fertilized as it travels down the Fallopian tube, within a few days it will implant itself in the spongy lining of the uterus. Throughout the pregnancy the mother's blood must carry a quantity of progesterone, for without it the uterus cannot maintain its contents and will abort the lining and the developing embryo. At first the *corpus luteum* provides sufficient progesterone, but as the placenta – the organ that transports food and oxygen to the foetus – develops in the uterine wall, it secretes progesterone in increasing amounts, and by the twelfth week of the pregnancy has taken over the task.

However, if there is no fertilization, the progesterone from the deteriorating *corpus luteum* is inadequate to maintain the endometrium. The endometrium then degenerates and menstruation occurs. The F S H from the pituitary again becomes dominant, and a new follicle, with its egg cell, begins to develop.

Menstruation is the process in which the lining of the uterus (endometrium), which is prepared anew each month as part of the cycle, is ejected. Menstrual fluid comes out through the vagina, and is a combination of these 'waste' products with some parts of blood – however, menstrual blood is not whole blood, because normally it contains no clotting agents that are present in whole blood. Menstruation requires from three to seven days a month, usually four or five. About a cup of menstrual fluid is produced over this period.

There is probably no topic in the world about which so little is generally known by ordinary people as menstruation. It has remained a tabooed topic of conversation long after most other aspects of sexuality have been brought into the open and discussed as a normal attribute of the human animal. Many of the primitive peoples of the world surround menstruation with taboos and rituals in order to control what they feel to be a highly dangerous state of affairs. In Europe and America we typically surround it with secrecy. Even today, medical scientists have done comparatively little in the study of menstruation and how to correct its difficulties when and if they appear, although this shortcoming is being alleviated.

Many situations in the life of a girl or a woman may interfere with the regularity of her menstrual periods. It usually takes a year or more for her periods to 'settle down' after menarche. Certainly it takes several months for them to become regular after the birth of a child, and usually the whole process of ovulation and menstruation is subject to irregularity and change at the time a girl begins an active sex life. Illnesses – fevers like malaria, intestinal upsets, or even serious constipation – can affect the cycle.

Female sexuality is geared to this cycle of menstruation and ovulation. The chemical rhythms of a woman's body are associated with it, and these chemical changes seem to be at the basis of the way some women feel and act at different times of the month. In some women, these chemical changes mean that the sexual urges are stronger at some points in the cycle than at others, and the points vary considerably from one woman to another. Some women have little or no discomfort during menstruation; they regulate their social and physical lives in accordance with it to only a slight degree. With other women, however, the hormone changes may not work as smoothly: either the rhythmic contractions of the muscular wall of the uterus may cause pain, or the endometrium may not be adequately broken down, so that pain results from its expulsion. Several delicate chemical and physical processes can go wrong, leading either to pain or to mental depression during menstruation. Worries and psychic states may also affect it. Thus some women may be either ill with headache and nervous jitters during their menstrual periods, or have a feeling of lassitude or of crankiness. These secondary symptoms, plus the effect of the pain itself, are often distressing to the other members of the family. A complete knowledge of what is occurring can, during these periods, allow the whole family to adjust to facts they understand.

During menstruation, women in the Western world wear either a sanitary pad or a tampon. A sanitary pad is a type of bandage which is placed over the vagina to absorb the flow of menstrual fluid. It is usually supported by a belt arrangement. The tampon is inserted into the vagina, and absorbs the fluid as it comes out of the uterus. Instructions in how to use these pads or tampons are to be found in the boxes in which they are sold.

The Female Life Cycle

Menarche, or first menstruation, usually occurs between the ages of eleven and fourteen in girls, but may be delayed in a few instances to as late as seventeen or eighteen. It is usually preceded by the enlargement of the breasts and the appearance of pubic hair and hair under the arms. There is no single line of development, and these events may take place in any order.

The menstrual cycle continues to operate in the normal woman for as much as thirty or thirty-five years. During that time, it will be altered if she becomes pregnant (as we shall see in Chapter 6), and may be altered by disease or other organic difficulties.

It used to be believed that the cycle ceased at whatever time the woman ran out of eggs. Today we know this is not true, but rather that the cessation of the cycle is a normal part of the ageing process. The ageing body normally produces smaller quantities of the hormones which control the cycle, and the result is that ultimately the cycle stops. This point in a woman's life is called menopause or change of life. The occurrence of menopause has nothing whatever to do with a woman's sexual desire or her capacity for sexual intercourse. It is, however, a trying experience for some women because of the change in their chemical metabolism. If there are psychological anxieties super-added to the physiological events, the difficulties can be very great, though again today, with increased knowledge, there is less difficulty experienced by most women at this stage of their lives than was the case in earlier times.

The menstrual cycle can, today, be continued artificially by providing the necessary hormones when the body no longer produces its own. It is said by some beauty experts that this process slows down the ageing process, but the full effects are not as yet known.

Ovulation may not occur during the first year or so after the initial appearance of menstruation, but it may – in fact, it may occur before. In the same way, the disappearance of menstruation at the time of menopause does not necessarily mean that ovulation stops at precisely the same time. Some women remain fertile for a couple of years after they cease to menstruate.

Female physiology is complicated – both in fact and by our lack of precise knowledge about it. Male physiology seems to be somewhat simpler, probably because hormonal periodicity and cycles are not an integral part of it. But that simplicity, too, may be an illusion resulting from ignorance of the details of body chemistry.

Chapter 4

Males

A greater proportion of the sexual equipment of the human male is on the outside of the body than is true of the female. It also was thought until recently to be a simpler mechanism. Probably such a comparison is meaningless, but there is one advantage of being male that is not purely a socially or culturally determined one: the male body does not undergo the kind of periodic chemical cycle which produces the ovulation and menstruation cycle in females. This is not to say that there are no chemical cycles of periodicity in the male, but if there are they have much less profound effect, and it is true that the physiologists know much less about them at the present time. This freedom from chemical – and hence mood – fluctuations is culturally useful to the male.

The chemical processes in the male genitals begin at the time of puberty and apparently continue until death, although they slow down their rate of activity as a normal part of the ageing process.

The Primary Sex Characteristics of Males

The purpose of the male sexual organs is to produce the sperm, which is analogous to the female egg, and to deposit it into female bodies. The various parts of the organs are the testicles, the *vas deferens*, the seminal vesicles, the prostate gland, and the penis.

The testicles. Sperm are created by the testicles, two oval organs that are enclosed in a bag of skin called the scrotum. The size of the testicles varies from about an inch to two inches along the long axis of the oval – the average seems to be a little less than one and a half inches. Size has nothing to do with the capacity to produce sperm, or, for that matter, with the size of the rest of the male genitals. Testicles are, long before birth, created from the same primitive tissue as are ovaries in the female. About two months before birth they descend into the scrotum, although sometimes they do not descend until several months after birth, and occasionally one or both testicles fail to descend at all.

It is important that at least one of the testicles be outside the body if the person is to be fertile, because even the internal temperature of the body is high enough to destroy the capacity to produce sperm. Indeed, heat that is scarcely uncomfortable to other parts of the body such as hands or feet can destroy the sperm-creating capacity for some weeks.

Each testicle (or testis) is a mass of tiny tubes, where the sperm are manufactured constantly. It used to be thought that sperm were created before birth, so that each male had only so many, and when they were gone, there would be no more. Today we know that they are manufactured constantly from puberty until death. Sperm leave the testicles and empty into a larger tube called the epididymis, which is coiled minutely around the top and back of each testicle. The epididymis, although it is coiled into a very small space, is almost twenty feet long. Sperm cells that are made in the tiny tubercles of the testicle are thought to be stored in the epididymis, but some physiologists dispute this view.

The vas deferens. Through the use of a swimming motion brought about by movement of the long tail on each sperm cell, the sperm make their way through the epididymis into a tube called the *vas deferens.* The *vas deferens* runs inside the pelvic bones and emerges over the top – the distance is about two inches, but the tube is coiled and is actually some six inches or more in length. This tube conducts the sperm to the seminal vesicles.

Figure 3. The Male Reproductive System

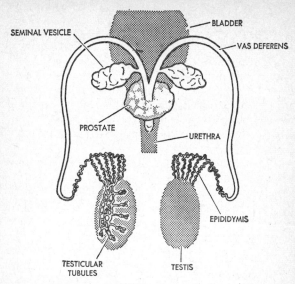

A. The route of the sperm into the urethra. The testis at left is shown in cross section.

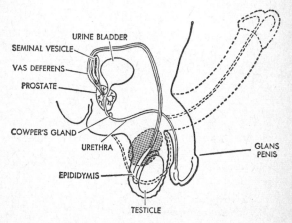

B. A side view of the male reproductive system.

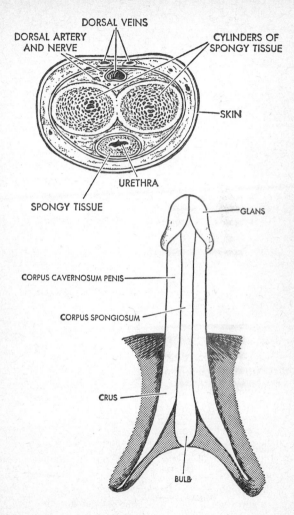

DORSAL VEINS

DORSAL ARTERY AND NERVE

CYLINDERS OF SPONGY TISSUE

SKIN

URETHRA

SPONGY TISSUE

GLANS

CORPUS CAVERNOSUM PENIS

CORPUS SPONGIOSUM

CRUS

BULB

C. A cross section of the penis.
D. The erect penis: ventral view.

The seminal vesicles. These two small organs lie just back of the prostate gland and secrete a substance which allows the sperm to move more freely. This seems to be the main place in which the sperm are stored.

The prostate gland. The prostate gland is a more or less round organ at the base of the urine bladder. The urethra, or urine tube, runs through it. The seminal vesicles are connected with it. The prostate manufactures a fluid in which the sperm can live and travel. This fluid is called semen. It is difficult to determine the exact size of the prostate of a living man and all measurements of it are only approximate – but it varies in the neighbourhood of an inch and a half across at the base. The prostate matures at sexual maturity, usually gets larger some time between the ages of forty and sixty, and then may become smaller again as the body ages.

The prostate gland also contains muscles for forcing the semen into the urethra at the climax stage of sexual excitement. At that time, the openings from the seminal vesicles are enlarged, and the openings of the prostate into the urethra are also enlarged, and about a teaspoon of semen is discharged into and through the penis.

The penis. The penis is the cylindrical organ which can be inserted into the vagina of a female. Through it the sperm are transported into the female's vagina. When the female's cervix settles into the pool of semen after intercourse, the situation is maximally favourable for survival and mobility to bring the sperm into contact with an egg.

The penis is made up of three cylinders of spongy tissue which fill with blood at the time of sexual stimulation and create erection of the penis. The smallest of these cylinders, called the spongy body (*corpus spongiosum*), contains the urethra, a tube which leads from the bladder and the prostate gland, up to the glans, or head of the penis. At the other end of the spongy body is another bulb of blood vessels and muscle which becomes engorged with blood during sexual excitation –

the expulsion of blood from this large bulb into the surrounding areas sets in motion the muscular contractions which constitute orgasm, and which move the seminal fluid from the prostate, along the urethra, to the outside of the body.

The size of the penis depends on the temperature of the environment, the general health of the man, and the state of sexual excitement. The length of the normal unerect or soft penis ranges from less than three inches to as much as five inches, with far the largest percentage being in the middle range. Smaller penises enlarge proportionally more at erection than do larger ones, according to recent studies, so that there tends to be less difference at erection than when they are not erect. The average length of the penis at erection is about six inches, but the range is from about five to about eight inches. The average breadth is a little over an inch and a half, and the average circumference a little over four inches.

Measurements of this sort are difficult to obtain, and not very important, except to a man himself at some stages of his life. The vagina of the female expands during sexual intercourse so as best to accommodate the specific penis, which means that the size of the penis has nothing to do with the sexual adequacy or capacity of the male.

Erections are common occurrences in the life of males of all ages. They start in tiny babies and go on until old age, although in some cases illness or psychological disturbances can create long periods in the life of a male in which he does not experience erection. Psychologists have recently found that normal males have erect penises during more than half of their dreaming time while asleep. This does not necessarily mean – and probably does not – that the content of the dream is sexual in nature. It may be, however, and one of the sure signs that a young man has reached puberty is that he may experience nocturnal emissions of semen, or wet dreams. This emission is a perfectly normal overflow of semen from the prostate, which occasionally empties itself automatically if no or few orgasms have occurred.

In past days, there were some strange beliefs about wet dreams and many fears were founded on these false beliefs. We now know that they are all superstitions and that wet dreams are a normal and perfectly harmless process.

Circumcision

At the time of birth, the skin continues as a sheath over the glans, or head of the penis. In many societies of the world this foreskin, or prepuce, is cut away in an operation called circumcision.

In modern Britain and America, most males born in hospitals are circumcised on the recommendation of the doctor, at the age of a day or two. There are some doctors and some psychiatrists who question the need or even the wisdom of performing this operation as a routine matter, but nevertheless it is commonly done. Many other Western societies, particularly the Scandinavian and Latin societies of Europe, do not practise non-medical circumcision. The reasons offered for circumcision, in those cultural traditions in which it is customary, range widely. It is sometimes said that it is easier to keep a circumcised penis clean, but it is certainly not difficult to keep an uncircumcised penis clean. It was formerly said in northern Europe and America that circumcision might reduce masturbation, but we know this is untrue because circumcision does not reduce sexual appetite – and, in any case, it is now known that masturbation, in itself, is not harmful. Several of the world's major religions and many tribal peoples perform circumcision as a religious offering. Islam and Judaism are the major examples. In this case, a portion of the creative organ is said to be offered to the Creator as a sacrifice, and also to gain fertility and as a prayer of gratitude.

Spermatogenesis

Like that of the female, the pituitary gland of the male secretes two sex hormones. One of these is FSH, the same hormone that triggers off ovulation in the female. It is also vital in creating sperm. The other pituitary hormone is called ICSH (interstitial cell-stimulating hormone). It is analogous to the LH of females, and it may be chemically the same substance, although some doubt about the precise chemical structure still exists. I C S H acts on the tiny bodies called the Leydig cells, which lie in the areas around the testicles and the epididymis, to make them secrete the male hormone testosterone,* which is necessary in the physiology of spermatogenesis and is the basis for the secondary masculine characteristics.

The process of spermatogenesis begins in the tubes of the testicles, where by a complicated chemical process, cells are split so that each one contains only one of each pair of genes of the individual. (Similarly, the egg in the female contains half of each pair.) Thereafter each sperm develops a tiny protein body with a long tail which allows it to 'swim' through the various male organs and, after implantation in the female, through the uterus and into the Fallopian tubes.

Doctors can count the number of sperm in the semen. Each ejaculation contains some 120,000,000 sperm. If the number goes much below 80,000,000 the man is usually sterile. It may, however, go up to three or more times the average, and sperm counts as high as 450,000,000 are unusual, but not rare. The higher the sperm count in the male, and the greater the motility of the sperm – that is, the better they can swim – then (if conditions are right in the female) the more likely it is that pregnancy will occur.

*All male hormones, including testosterone, are called androgens. Female hormones are called oestrogens. The adrenal glands of both sexes produce large quantities of both androgens and oestrogens. Oestrogens in males cannot be assigned a specific function, at the present time at least; androgens are the triggering mechanism, in both sexes, for the physical conditions which both males and females feel as sexual tension. Although adrenal androgens can be converted into testosterone, the amount of androgens in males is vastly increased at puberty by the supply of testosterone from the testes, which promotes development of the secondary sex characteristics. Scientists have discovered in the last few years that the mammalian foetus develops as a female, no matter what its genetic structure, unless androgen is supplied from the male foetus. In birds and reptiles the situation is reversed, and all the animals develop as males unless the change is made by oestrogen early in the foetal period.

Male Sexuality

It is important to note that sexual feelings in males are aroused at different rates and by lesser stimulus than in females. This fact does not mean that the sexual drive in the male is stronger, but only that full arousal in the male may be a matter of only a few seconds, whereas it is almost always a matter of several minutes in the female.

Young males should not think that females are uninterested in sex, but they certainly should not think that girls' feelings work like their own. And young females should certainly know that men were 'created that way', and *not* think that they are all socially or personally inept or clumsy.

We should also admit frankly that since a greater proportion of the male sexual organs are on the outside of the body, they are subjected to a more or less constant stimulation from clothes and changes in bodily position. Men are aware of their genitals in the course of a large proportion of their activities. I do not of course mean that women are not constantly aware of being women, as men are aware of being men, but rather that male genitals must be protected during violent exercise, and that males are constantly aware of this need to protect themselves. A woman's need for protection is not based so fundamentally and primarily on her genitals – but most modern girls prefer to wear brassieres when they are active, and perhaps can see the analogy to male feelings.

Thus, it is often difficult for girls and even adult women to understand the constancy of the sexual pressure on males, just as it is sometimes difficult for males to understand that the females once aroused have very strong sexual urges. Like almost anything else, however, knowledge about these matters makes it possible for people to understand one another and their actions and theri drives.

Chapter 5

The Facts About Sexual Intercourse

It is astonishing but nevertheless true that only in the years after 1950 has the physiology of sexual intercourse come to be thoroughly understood. It was, after all, only in the 1930s that physiologists first saw a human egg. It was scarcely thirty years before that that the full details of the anatomy (let alone the physiology) of the male sexual organs was investigated. And as recently as 1966 it was pointed out by M. J. Sherfey, a psychiatrist who had made a thorough investigation, that there was not available in any book of anatomy an adequate description of the musculature and nerve physiology of the clitoris.

The physiology of sex seems to be one of the last major areas – certainly it is the most recent – to be thoroughly investigated by scientists. Surely no other part of the anatomy or no other physiological functions have ever been so surrounded with shame and superstition, making even our scientists afraid to look.

This chapter is about the physiology of sexual intercourse, and something about the way in which our language deals with it. I have made every attempt to avoid moral colouring – that is the subject of the second half of the book. After all, psychic differences in the way you feel it or feel about it may inhibit some of the functions of the glands and muscles, but they cannot change them otherwise.

Sexual Intercourse

Sexual intercourse is the generic term given to the activity in which the penis is inserted into the vagina and in which, after a series of back and forward thrusting movements, the penis ejects

51

Love, Sex and Being Human

seminal fluid into the vagina. In most human societies, sexual intercourse is preceded by some form of 'sex play'. This is, however, a cultural addition to the somatic basis of intercourse, and it may be absent. Similarly, intercourse may be followed by sex play, and may not be – again, it is a cultural addition. Since foreplay and afterplay are cultural matters, which change from one society to another, and from one historical period to another, they will not be discussed further here – any good marriage manual covers the subject in detail.

There are several words, with different detailed meanings,that can be applied to sexual intercourse. Some of them at least should be known. The word 'copulation' comes from the Latin word meaning to join or unite; this word, when applied to sexual intercourse, is more or less morally neutral. The same can be said for the words 'coitus' and 'coition', both of which come from the Latin word meaning to go together. Doctors usually use the word 'coitus' when they discuss human sexual intercourse.

Other words have a moral element added to them. 'Fornication' means voluntary sexual intercourse between unmarried persons. If either or both of the partners are married, but not to one another, their intercourse is 'adultery'. If the act is not voluntary on the part of one partner, it may be 'rape'. Sometimes in American legal language the word 'fornication' is used to include all non-marital sexual intercourse, including adultery. The word 'adultery' is sometimes used for fornication because to some it seems less 'vulgar' in sound.

There are also several vivid, short Anglo-Saxon words which are even yet not usable in what is commonly considered to be polite society. Most persons who speak English know these words by the time they are out of primary school, if not well before. The difficulty in these Anglo-Saxon words does not result from their sexual meaning. Rather, they are words in which sex and aggression merge. We have no simple and abrupt words or even any swear words for aggression in English. It is the combination of aggression with sex that is unacceptable in the drawing room.

It might be easier to describe the male and female experiences

52

of sexual intercourse separately. But such a description would fail to give the picture of complementarity. Sexual intercourse is a social act. Although it is experienced in two different minds and bodies, it is nevertheless a single activity. For this reason, I will describe the total activity and give, at the same time, the occurrences in each partner.

Masters and Johnson, in their classic but highly technical book, *Human Sexual Response*, have divided the act of human sexual intercourse into four phases, stating forthrightly that they have found this division convenient for explanation, and that the sex act is not an undisputable 'series' of 'events'. They might have used three phases (combining their excitement and plateau), or they might have used five (by subdividing any one of the phases, probably plateau). Yet there are natural criteria (more marked in the female than the male) which led them to make the sensible division that they made. They called these four stages (1) excitement, (2) plateau, (3) orgasm, and (4) resolution. The names were chosen because the first can be reversed without undue difficulty, the second can be prolonged by choice and control, the third is a technical term for muscle spasms that are involuntary once they have begun, and the fourth 'resolves' the organism to its pre-excitement state.

Each of the four phases is more likely to be quickly achieved and more quickly finished by the male than by the female. The aim of all experienced and considerate lovers is for the partners to go through the phases together – most people think that the act is more pleasurable when this is the case. However, it is surely true that complete concert is not always achieved by any couple, and is never achieved by some.

It should also be remembered throughout the description that human sexuality and response involves the entire body and not merely the genitals, although our description will centre on the genitals.

Excitement phase. In the male the initial response to sexual excitation is erection of the penis. The erection is usually involuntary and can be fully achieved in from three to eight seconds, though it is in some degree possible to inhibit the erection, especially after the age of twenty or so. The time required for an erection usually increases with age after about forty, but even then erection can still be achieved very quickly by most males. The erection is created when nerve endings at the base of the penis cause the veins that carry blood away from the penis to contract, thus engorging the spongy tissues of the three penile columns with blood.

Females in the initial phases of sexual excitement have an equally involuntary response in that tiny pores within the vagina begin to release a slippery liquid lubricant, and the vagina begins to get bigger. The lubrication usually appears in from ten to thirty seconds. After the age of forty this process also may be slowed a little.

At this phase, sexual excitement can easily be stopped. However, if it continues, the next phase in both sexes is the engorgement of the genitalia by blood – in addition, of course, to the blood which has already created the erection in the male. This area to be filled with blood is much more extensive in the female than it is in the male, and the process of the congestion of blood takes several minutes and cannot be hurried: physiologically a woman cannot speed up the time required for her to go through the excitement stage. In males, the engorgement at this stage is in the penile bulb and the surrounding areas; since the area is smaller than in the female, it can be completed very much more quickly. In the male, the engorgement also leads to thickening of the skin of the scrotum, with the result that the testicles are elevated towards the body. In an almost precisely analogous way, the *labia majora* of the female are elevated so that they separate, and the *labia minora* may increase in size two or three times. As excitement proceeds in the male, the testicles increase in size, sometimes as much as fifty per cent. The inner two thirds of the female's vagina expands and extends so that several centimetres are added to the length of the vaginal barrel, which also becomes wider.

It is during the excitement phase that some of the non-genital physical reactions begin to appear. In about eighty per cent of women, and in somewhat more than half of men, the nipples become erect and hard. A rush of blood to the skin may provide what is called the 'sex flush', which usually starts on the chest and spreads to the neck and forehead, and sometimes, especially in women, also to the belly and the thighs. Not all people exhibit this sex flush, and apparently nobody does on all occasions. Perspiration may appear – independent of the heat of the room or the physical effort expended.

Plateau phase. During the early plateau phase of sexual tension, more extensive changes are taking place in the female than in the male. In the late plateau phase the situation is reversed.

In the female, the cervix, or opening of the uterus, rises at the same time that the vaginal barrel is distended further. This forms a sack-like area in the depth of the vagina where the semen will be deposited. At the same time, the engorgement of the outer third of the vagina increases, so that area actually becomes smaller in diameter. Masters and Johnson have called this the 'orgasmic platform'.

Meanwhile, the penis may again increase in circumference at the ridge of the glans; the testicles are brought up tight against the body, sometimes, in fact, being taken into the body in the pubic area just beneath the skin.

In many persons, both men and women, there are colour changes in the sex organs at this time due to changes in the arterial and venous blood supplies. In both sexes there are mucous secretions in this phase – from the Cowper's glands of the male and from the Bartholin's glands of the female. These secretions create the alkaline environment necessary for sperm to live long enough to achieve impregnation.

Orgasm. Orgasm is similar in the two sexes in that it begins when the distension caused by the congestion of blood reaches a point at which the surrounding muscles are caused to contract vigorously; they are the same muscles in the two sexes. The muscular contraction has the effect of forcing out some of the congested blood, and with the male also the seminal fluid. It is the contraction of the muscles and the rushing out of fluids that create the sensations of orgasm. With the female the orgasm is the displacement of a relatively large amount of blood from the congested areas to nearby areas; with the male the orgasm involves the displacement of a relatively small amount of blood from the smaller congested areas, and also the expulsion of the semen. There are more contractions in the female than the male – more fluid must be moved. The most intense period of male orgasm lasts three to four seconds, female five to six seconds.

The first event of the male orgasm involves the muscular contraction and spasms of the *vas deferens*, the seminal vesicles and the prostate. This process moves the semen into the portion of the urethra closest to the prostate gland. The second event of the orgasm, which occurs about three seconds later, is the rhythmical expansion and contraction of the bulb of the penis, and of the muscles surrounding it. The contractions take place about every .8 seconds and provide a considerable expulsive pressure for the semen, which emerges in spurts. The sensation is concentrated in the penis, and many men are unaware of the internal contractions or those of the muscles surrounding the bulb.

The female orgasm begins with what has been described as a sensation of suspension that emanates from contraction of the uterus, followed immediately by a single thrust of feeling that spreads from the clitoris upward into the pelvis. The second event is a 'suffusion of warmth' throughout the body. The third is an involuntary contraction of the vagina, sometimes felt throughout the lower pelvis. Some women distinguish first the contraction, then a throbbing, which would make four events or sensational phases.

The Resolution Phase. The resolution phase is the period just after orgasm, when the genitals and other body parts return to the pre-excitement condition: the cervix descends into the semen pool, the vagina contracts; the penis becomes flaccid, and the testicles return to the original size and position. It has been observed by Masters and Johnson, as a matter of fact but not

Table 1–Phases of Sexual Response

	Excitement	Plateau	Orgasm	Resolution
♀	(several minutes to several hours)	(3 minutes to 30 seconds)	(3–15 seconds)	(10–15 minutes; if no orgasm, ½ day or more)
	Nipple erection	Apparent retraction of clitoris as hood is engorged with blood	3–15 contractions in lower vagina	Return to normal condition
	Clitoris enlarges	Enlarged labia gap	contractions of uterus	Relaxation of organs; cervix thus immersed in seminal pool left in vagina
	Increase in size of *labia minora*	Slight contractions of uterus in some cases		
	Cervix rises	Increased vaginal secretion		
	Vaginal secretion			
♂	(10 seconds to several hours)			
	Erection of penis	Additional vaso-congestion of *glans penis*	Muscular contractions of internal, then external organs every .8 seconds for 3 or 4 spasms, then irregularly and weakly	Detumescence of penis, time depending on how long the plateau was maintained
	Thickening of skin of scrotum; testicles thus elevated	Testicles elevated to contact perineum; testicles increase in size	Ejaculation of semen	Size and position of testicles returns to normal

57

totally explained, that the longer the plateau phase has lasted, the longer the resolution phase requires. Generally speaking, however, the resolution phase is shorter for the male than for the female.

Sexual Capacity

The female is capable of several orgasms in a much shorter time than is the male. M. J. Sherfey, the psychiatrist and physiologist, explains this on the basis of the more extensive areas of the female which have been congested with blood, so that blood expelled by the orgasm can return almost immediately, whereas replacement takes longer in the male. Most males must return to the excitement phase before they are again brought back to the plateau phase and are capable of a second orgasm. Females can experience multiple orgasms – half a dozen is not uncommon, and the counted number according to both Masters and Sherfey has gone to over fifty, to create what Sherfey has called 'satiation-in-insatiation'.

Nobody knows the sexual capacity of a human being over a time, because it is always affected by social, cultural, and psychic considerations – it may be increased and it may be decreased by many physical and psychic stimuli. Sexual intercourse may be had several times a day for relatively short periods, and it may be dispensed with entirely for longer or shorter periods. Alfred Kinsey found, some quarter of a century ago, that the average number of orgasms was about three a week, or a little over, for males and females, but like all averages, it encompasses vast differences, some persons having very few orgasms, and others as many as several a day.

It should again be pointed out that the facts in this chapter are primarily biological, with some cultural asides. I shall consider the psychic and the further cultural and social factors of human sexual intercourse in later parts of this book. It should also be noted that there has been no mention of techniques or positions in sexual intercourse. I think that such information should be known and understood by everyone, and that it should be readily available. It is readily available in any good marriage manual. I also think it is quite another topic from that of the present book, which is a book of biological, psychological, and cultural information rather than a 'how to' book.

Chapter 6

The Physiology of Conception

We have already seen that a woman produces one or, on a few occasions, more eggs per month, and that they enter into the Fallopian tubes from the ovaries. We have also seen that the male ejaculates about a teaspoon of semen which contains millions of sperm.

The semen is received into a hollow place in the back of the barrel of the vagina, where it forms what Masters and Johnson have called the 'semen pool'. During intercourse, the opening of the uterus, which is called the cervix, has been raised; as sexual excitation resolves itself and the woman's internal genitalia settle back into position, the cervix is immersed in the semen pool. The sperm swim in the seminal fluid, and some of them enter the opening of the cervix and find their way into the uterus and on up into the Fallopian tubes. A high concentration of sperm is necessary for one sperm to be successful in breaking through the covering, or soft 'shell' of the egg (called the *zona pellucida*, or 'transparent zone').

At this moment, when the cell contained in the sperm and that contained in the egg unite, conception takes place. This is not the place to go into details of genes, chromosomes, and the principles of heredity. That subject is extremely complex, and belongs in a special study in biology. Here it is important for us to know that the only cells in the human body which are not complete cells are those of the egg and the sperm; one of each is necessary to create a complete cell. The cell which is created at the time of conception is the cell from which all of the bodily cells of the future human being arise. In short, a child gets half of his genes from his mother and half from his father. The sex of the child is determined by whether an X chromosome or a Y chromosome, as they are called, is contained in the sperm which is finally successful in fertilizing the egg. The sex of the child is determined by the sperm cell, not by the egg, and it would seem to be a matter of absolute chance. That last statement would be questioned by some authorities, who claim that the chemical environment of the female – or even her age – influence the likelihood of success of one type over the other type of sperm, but our knowledge in these matters is scanty at best.

The fertilized egg is, then, a single cell. Mammalian eggs can afford to be extremely small because the nourishment for the young does not have to be stored in the yolk, as is the case with birds and reptiles, whose eggs must contain sufficient nutrient for the new organism until the time it hatches. The extremely miniature scale on which human conception takes place can be realized when we know that the individual sperm is only 1/500 of an inch long. The egg can just be seen with the naked eye, but is small enough to pass easily through the Fallopian tubes, which internally measure little more than the thickness of a hair.

Yet the new cell contains several tens of thousands of genes. We do not know the precise number, but we do know that each nucleus – that is, the nucleus of the sperm and that of the egg – contains at least fifteen thousand and perhaps a good many more. In the last few years, genes have been found to contain chemical 'instructions' as to the nature of the new cells that are to form in the new human being.

The combination of the genes and chromosomes of the two nuclei is complete about thirty minutes or so after the sperm has broken into the egg. In this short time, all of a person's physical characteristics and undoubtedly many of his mental and psychic characteristics are determined. Immediately after the formation of the new cell, the processes of cellular division begin. With the combination of the genes from the father and the mother, a new individual has been created. With the first division, he begins to grow and mature.

On the third or fourth day after fertilization, the tiny cell cluster, still within the shell-like *zona pellucida*, has completed the journey through the Fallopian tube and has entered the uterus.

The first few days it is in the uterus, or womb, the fertilized cell floats about in the watery substance contained in the womb, and eventually settles into the sponge-like endometrium, which now, instead of being expelled as menstrual fluid, is allowed to continue to build up as the foetus develops. It is probable that the sixth or seventh day sees the nutrients in the yolk of the human egg almost exhausted. The new cell cluster nestles into the spongy lining of the uterus and grows a set of 'roots' called *villi,* which hold it fast to the wall of the uterus, and which seem also to be used for the taking in of nourishment.

By the ninth day, the embryo has been well implanted. The rate of the duplication of cells is vastly increased, and the specialization of cells begins. We shall continue the story of life before birth in Chapter 8. Before that, however, we should examine the ways in which conception is inhibited or in which it can be avoided.

Chapter 7

Contraception

Nature overdoes everything. Indeed, everything that is not over-done in nature may fail to survive if living conditions become even slightly unfavourable. Creatures such as fish produce tens or even hundreds of thousands of young each season in order that a few of the next generation may survive to the age of reproduction. Most reptiles must produce hundreds of young; dogs and rabbits must produce litters at a time.

It is true that human beings need to produce only a few off-spring to assure the next generation. But it is also true that to assure these few, nature has overdone the biology of reproduction and the sex drive in man. We have seen that each ejaculation of semen contains hundreds of millions of sperm, and that each ovary could be capable of producing tens of thousands of eggs.

Today, because of improvements in health and culture, a greater proportion of the human beings who are conceived live to be born than ever before, and a far greater proportion who are born live to reproduce. When so large a proportion of people live to reproduce, the reproduction rate is vastly increased and the population grows with radical new speed.

If the growth of the population is not checked, it will destroy the very world which it developed – or at least make it unin-habitable by human beings. All thinking people, all religious and political groups, agree that the world's population growth must be checked.

At the same time, they are also coming to realize that the non-reproductive benefits of sexuality are to be retained. Only a small proportion of our sexual drive is required to assure reproduction. The rest must be either utilized for other personal and social purposes or suppressed. Complete suppression of the sex drive for extended periods of time has never been successful for many people.

The goal, then, is on the one hand to achieve an adequate replacement of the population at the same time that we avoid the dangers of overpopulation. On the other hand we must see that the sex drive, as an integral part of our personalities, continues to inform our emotions and enrich our experience of life.

To achieve both these purposes the proportion of sexual acts that lead to reproduction must be reduced. Most thinking people of every civilized society, some of them organized into large groups, are concerned with contraception, which means 'against conception', or interference with conception. While it is true that some of these people are organized to *prevent* contraception, their number is daily becoming smaller. Contraception is a part of living in the present and the future which is being and will be accepted as a commonplace.

Theories and Means of Contraception

It is obvious that as long as the sperm does not reach the egg, or the fertilized egg does not settle into the lining of the uterus, pregnancy cannot occur. There are several points in the involved biological process of conception at which contraceptive principles can be applied. In explaining the various methods that can be used for contraception, I have arranged them in rough order following the normal processes of conception:

1. The sperm are not allowed to enter the vagina
a. under any conditions.
b. on specific days of the menstrual cycle, i.e., during and immediately after ovulation.
2. Having entered the vagina, the sperm are not allowed to live.
3. The sperm enter the vagina, but are kept from entering the uterus and the Fallopian tubes.

4. The hormonal balance of the animals is changed so that no egg is present or else no sperm are present.

5. The uterus is kept open with a mechanical device which upsets the timing of the menstrual cycle in such a way as to prevent conception.

We shall take up these methods one at a time, remembering that some of them might be put under more than one of these headings.

1. *The sperm are not allowed to enter the vagina.* It is often said that the surest contraceptive is abstinence from sexual intercourse. Certainly this is so, but it is not a practicable method for many people during many years of their adult lives.

It is possible, however, to practise a partial or timed abstinence, called 'rhythm'. We have seen that the length of life of the egg in the Fallopian tubes is probably no more than thirty hours unless it is fertilized. Obviously, if there is abstinence during that period, no pregnancy can occur. There are tremendous practical difficulties in the way, however. All sorts of physical influences can change the precise days of ovulation of a woman. Ovulation should occur about halfway between menstrual periods, but it is well known that sickness, travel, emotional upset, changes in the amount of sexual activity (particularly those that follow on initiation of full sexual activity, which usually happens at marriage), and many other factors can affect the timing of the menstrual cycle. It is, moreover, unknown how long sperm can live in the vagina and uterus of a woman. This depends, of course, on the chemical composition of the lubricants in the vagina and the fluids in the uterus. Certainly it may vary from as little as five minutes to as long as several days. Rhythm is the least effective method of contraception of those used.

There are two other methods by which sperm are kept out of the vagina. One is that the male withdraws before ejaculation. This is called *coitus interruptus*, and demands a great deal of emotional and physical control if it is to be practised successfully. Because it interrupts or stops the course of orgasm, it will never be popular: it requires very great concentration and resolve.

The penis may be covered by a sheath of very fine rubber or fish membranes – several other fine membranes have been or are now being used in various parts of the world. The sheath, called a condom, catches the semen as it is ejaculated, thereby preventing its being laid down in the seminal pool within the vagina. In Britain, condoms can be bought at chemists'. Condoms have the disadvantage that they reduce the sensation for both sexes.

2. *The sperm are not allowed to remain alive.* It is possible to change the chemical composition of the vaginal environment so as to kill the sperm on contact. Sperm require a slightly alkaline environment. If the environment is changed to a slightly acidic one they will perish. It may be physically dangerous to try to create an acid environment in the vagina with any chemicals other than those sold specifically for the purpose, or those sug- gested by a doctor. It is possible to purchase (also at chemists') vaginal jellies and creams that are made for this purpose. Vaginal foams contain the same mildly acidic spermatocide and also create a foamy environment in which the sperm are unable to swim. These must all be applied before intercourse.

In the old days, some women tried by 'douching' to wash the semen out of the vagina immediately after intercourse. A few still do. The effectiveness of douching is almost none.

3. *The sperm are kept out of the uterus and Fallopian tubes.* Another way to avoid conception is to cover the cervix, or entry into the uterus, in such a way that the sperm cannot enter it in order to swim into the uterus and Fallopian tubes. This is achieved by a rubber diaphragm, stretched over a spring frame, which fits into the vagina and is lodged against the pelvic bone in such a way as to cover the cervix. Diaphragms have to be fitted by a physician on the basis of individual measurements if they are to be effective. They are usually combined with spermatocidal jellies or creams during use. They can be inserted several hours before intercourse and remain effective.

4. *Pills to change the hormonal balance.* The production of

eggs by the female can be controlled and, indeed, prevented by the administration by mouth (or by injection) of hormones which change the course of the menstrual cycle. The hormones inhibit ovulation completely, so that no egg is present to be fertilized.

It is also possible, through drugs, to prevent the manufacture of sperm in the male. Most doctors consider it dangerous. The sperm count of a man can (without influencing the production of seminal fluid) be lowered to the point where pregnancy cannot occur, but the drugs in their present state of development are unpredictable. It is not known what side effects may ensue, or whether or not full capacity to create sperm can ever be regained. The hormonal drugs given to males to stop the manufacture of sperm work over a period of many months, or even years.

The hormonal drugs presently given to women as contraceptives work only for a single menstrual cycle – indeed, when women are withdrawn from the drug, fertility is enhanced. Most of these drugs are taken as pills and most are taken every day for twenty of the twenty-eight days of the menstrual cycle. The hormone progesterone inhibits ovulation – particularly when it is combined with oestrogens. All the contraceptive pills in use at the moment are a combination of these two hormones. In one method, called 'combined', both are taken during the entire twenty days. In the other, called 'sequential', estrogen is taken for ten days and then progesterone for ten days (sometimes the number of days on oestrogen is increased). It would seem that the combined method is almost 100 per cent effective; the sequential method a little less so.

The long-term effects of artificially changing the rhythm of the hormonal cycle in women are not known. What is true is that every month the woman goes through a speeded-up hormonal experience of pregnancy and delivery, rather than a menstrual cycle. The late Gregory Pincus, who was the leader in the discovery and development of oral contraceptives, stated specifically in *Science* in 1966 that 'Except for clear and expected hormonal actions of progestins and oestrogens, I know of no scientifically valid demonstration of significant pathological effects of their use in contraceptive doses and regimens.' About the same time, the editors of the *Ladies' Home Journal* brought together an impressive array of medical and scientific opinion that accentuated our ignorance about the matter, as well as case histories in which illness and even death seem to have resulted from side effects – blood clotting, eye difficulties and loss of hair have been reported. It is certain that no woman with a history of endocrinal problems should ever take the pill. There is also some doubt about the long-term effects on the pituitary of the inhibition of production of luteinizing hormone.

The only facts seem to be that the demand for birth-control pills is very great and that vast pressures are put on doctors to prescribe them. The efficiency of the pill is the greatest of any known method but the long-term chemical effect is unknown; many authorities are worried about it.

There are also surgical ways, called 'sterilization', of preventing ovulation and spermatogenesis. The Fallopian tubes can be severed or tied off surgically in such a way that eggs cannot descend through them or sperm ascend into them. However, in the normal processes of healing, new pathways are occasionally created so that even such surgery is not absolutely sure. Sterilization of women is usually not reversible – the reversal is a difficult operation and is often not successful. In the male, it is possible either to sever or to plug the *vas deferens* so that sperm cannot get from the testicles to the prostate. This is a minor operation and can sometimes, but certainly not always, be reversed. It is also not always successful – there are case histories in which even a second operation did not bring about sterilization.

Sterilization does not affect a person's capacity for or enjoyment of sexual intercourse, except insofar as the knowledge that no children can be conceived on any occasion sometimes reduces (but sometimes enhances) enjoyment. Sterilization is illegal in most states of the United States, except for medical reasons. Even in those places where it is not illegal, most doctors will not perform the operation. They consider that other modes of contraception are workable and are not subject to the same psychological side effects (which sterilization has in many cases) or the same possibilities of long-run regret.

5. *Upsetting the ovulation-menstrual cycle mechanically.* Whereas the pill upsets the cycle of ovulation and menstruation by chemical means, and sterilization attempts by surgery to prevent the presence of the egg at the time in the cycle it would normally appear, it is also possible to achieve a similar end mechanically. Doctors can insert a plastic loop, coil, or ring into the opening of the cervix, which thus prevents its closing. This loop, usually of nylon, is called an 'intra-uterine device', or I.U.D. We do not at present know exactly how the device works or why it is contraceptive, but in fact it is almost as efficient as the pill. It has been said that circulating air through the uterus may interfere with the lodgement of the egg in the endometrium, but nobody knows for sure that this is true. It has also been said that the presence of the device so speeds up the process of ovulation and expulsion of the egg that there is very little time for its fertilization and none for implantation, but we also do not know whether that is true. At the present writing, the physiological changes worked by the intra-uterine device are being extensively studied in laboratory animals, and we should learn how it works before long. Many gynaecologists will not insert I.U.D.s because many years ago, with quite different devices made of metal, a number of infections occurred. With the new plastic materials, these difficulties have been removed.

I.U.D.s are expelled by some women – about twenty per cent has been the usual estimate. However, after the birth of at least one child most women can retain them. A thread is usually left emerging from the cervix so that a woman can determine whether the device is still in place. I.U.D.s may be painful for a few days or as much as a month. It may take a month or two for the menstrual periods to settle back to regularity. However, once the adjustment has been made, the intra-uterine device is permanent, painless, and totally undetectable. It can be easily removed by a physician, and the woman's normal fertility immediately restored.

Objections to Contraception

Some people object to some methods of contraception on personal grounds. It is true that the only methods that never alter the sensations are the oral contraceptives and the intra-uterine device. However, many object to the oral contraceptives because they change the hormone cycle, and the long-term effect of such alteration is not known. Most men object to condoms because they always reduce the sensation for him and usually also for his partner. A few people – both men and women – can detect the presence of diaphragms, though they are not uncomfortable. Some say that the jellies, creams, and foams change the texture of the lubrication, and therefore the sensation. Most people, however, do not find either diaphragms or foams objectionable, either because they cannot detect a difference, or because the slight difference is not unpleasant.

Some groups of people object to one or more methods of contraception on doctrinal grounds. By far the largest group to take such a position is the Roman Catholic Church. Even they do not object to the idea of contraception, but only to specific methods. The only method that the Church now approves of is the least efficient – the rhythm method. Their position, however, is being considered and it may change in the future.

Natural Sterility

It should be noted in closing this chapter that although the overwhelming number of human beings are fertile – that is, capable of producing children – a few are not. Infertility probably does not affect them in any other way, including their sex lives. Such people are called sterile. Most sterile people are unprepared to discover their condition, because all of us are brought up to expect to be parents. Thus sterility usually comes as a surprise, and can lead to great emotional upset.

Modern medical practice has made good progress in understanding and treating sterility, making it possible for many formerly sterile persons who want children to have them, and for

Table 2–Means of Contraception and Their Effectiveness

Method	Procedure	Reliability	Side Effects or Other Disadvantages
1a. Withdrawal	Male withdraws penis from vagina before ejaculation.	Unsafe – semen may escape into vagina before ejaculation	Unnatural interruption of intercourse leaves couple tense and unsatisfied.
b. Condom	During intercourse penis is covered with a cap of rubber, animal intestine, or fish membrane.	Fairly safe – faulty rubber may rip and allow semen to spill into vagina	Some couples feel the sensations are decreased.
c. Rhythm	Woman determines when ovulation occurs in her cycle, avoids intercourse at that time.	Unsafe – great risk of pregnancy	Cycle is easily disrupted, invalidating woman's calculations. Few women have absolutely regular periods.
2. Spermicidal jelly or foam	It is injected into vagina with special applicator before intercourse. Foam reduces mobility of sperm. Acidity kills sperm.	Unsafe – sperm may survive in vaginal crevices unreached by jelly or foam	A few women show allergic reactions to jelly or cream – local rash or irritation.
3. Diaphragm	Before intercourse, woman places rubber cap in vagina to wall off the cervix, preventing sperm from entering. Usually used with a spermicidal jelly.	Less than 1% of users report failure if properly fitted and cared for	A few women are unwilling or unable to learn to insert diaphragm. It demands a certain amount of planning ahead. Otherwise foreplay may have to be interrupted for insertion.
4. Hormone pills	Woman takes daily pills to stop ovulation.	Nearly totally reliable when used exactly as directed	Some users suffer nausea, legcramps, breakthrough bleeding, breast soreness, or other unpleasant side effects. Some doctors feel current rise in deaths from thrombosis due to pill. Medical effects not fully known.
5. Intra-uterine device (I.U.D.)	Gynaecologist inserts loop into uterus; it can be removed by any gynaecologist when woman wants to become pregnant.	Almost total	About 80% of those inserted are retained; some women find I.U.D. to be painful and have it removed, though in most the pain is not severe, and disappears totally within a month.

many couples to be able to conceive who could not have done so without such medical help.

Finally, two important points: no recognized group of people today wants to deny the privileges and joys of parenthood to any normal individual. They do claim, however, that it is possible to be just as much a parent with two or three children as with a dozen. Perhaps, some argue, you can even be a better parent because each child can have more parental time and attention. Contraception and control of the total population, and the quality of family life, as well as opportunity for experiencing the full range of one's sexuality, all come together in this question. It is one of the most important questions in today's world.

Further, few groups today still want to deny the pleasure and security of normal sexuality to those who are physically and socially in a position to enjoy them. Contraception is important to them, because throughout much of their lives, freedom from fear of pregnancy can give an important psychological boost to the relationship.

Chapter 8

Life Before Birth

Although in the Western world we count our age from the date of birth, we nevertheless realize that life begins not with birth, but with conception. What Westerners are counting is only the age of the child as a social creature, not its total age as a living organism.

The First Six Months of Life

From the time that the fertilized human egg imbeds itself into the lining of the uterus at the age of six or seven days until its birth sometime between 265 and 280 days after conception, the human individual grows far more than in any other comparable time span during life. The one cell which was created at the time of conception turns into over two billion cells at the time of birth.

The new organism is called an embryo from the time of conception to the time that its species is recognizable, which in human beings is at about the seventh week. After that, the organism is called a foetus until the time of its birth.

Perhaps the most important thing about the human foetus is that after the first few weeks, it reacts to outside stimulus. The influence of pre-natal environments is extremely important in determining what the individual reactions will be. We do not yet know as much as we ought to know about the nature of the pre-natal environment and its influence on the physical and mental health of the eventual adult. We do know that X-rays, many drugs – including nicotine – and other substances have some adverse influence on the formation and growth of the embryo and foetus.

Today pediatricians and psychiatrists are of the opinion that some qualities of personality may result from the specific environment of the pre-natal life. The chemical aspects of this environment are dependent on the health and emotional welfare of the mother during pregnancy. However, it is not now possible – and will probably remain difficult or impossible – to distinguish the effects of pre-natal experience from the natural genetic endowment of the individual. It is a matter of fact, however, that the health and mental attitudes of the mother may be reflected in the child. Illness and nervous tension of their mothers seem to have an adverse effect on babies, before as well as after birth.

The most characteristic aspect of mammalian reproduction is the presence of a placenta. Branching tissues from the embryo interlaced with the spongy endometrium form this astonishing and versatile organ. The blood of the child flows into and out of the placenta through arteries and veins in the umbilical cord. The carbon dioxide produced by the child's body is exchanged in the placenta for oxygen from the mother's blood stream. Food substances in the mother's blood are carried across the placental tissues into the child's bloodstream; the child's urea is transferred back to the mother's blood, from which it is removed by her kidneys. Thus the placenta functions in the unborn child as the lungs, kidneys, and digestive system will function after birth.

The whole blood of the child never mixes directly with the mother's blood, and never leaves the self-enclosed set of veins and arteries, which includes some of those of the placenta, those of the umbilical cord, and those of the child's body. However, some of the constituents of the blood are exchanged. This fact explains the pathologies that result when the child inherits from the father a type of blood that is incompatible with the blood of the mother.*

*One of the many aspects of human blood that can vary, through inheritance, among individuals is the so-called 'Rhesus factor'. If a woman without the Rhesus factor conceives a child who has inherited its father's Rhesus factor, and the Rhesus substance passes through the placental membranes into the mother's bloodstream, antibodies are developed in her blood. When these antibodies enter the child's bloodstream – again, through the placental membranes – they damage the child's red blood cells and

The placenta relays antibodies from the mother's blood, making the foetal child immune to many diseases. It is the maturing and ageing of the placenta which triggers the changes in hormonal balance that lead to the processes of birth. At the time of birth, the placenta weighs about a pound, and it is discarded, with the amniotic membranes, as the 'afterbirth'.

We know a great deal about the day-by-day development of the human embryo, its growth into a foetus, and its ultimate birth as a child. The limbs appear as tiny buds on the embryo when it is less than a month old. At that time, the embryo is completely formed, although it is less than half an inch in length. The heart is usually beating a few days before the end of the first month of life. At this time the baby is enclosed in a sort of bag called the amniotic sac, in a completely liquid environment. He will remain in this sac until it breaks at birth or a little before and exposes the child to air for the first time.

By the seventh week, the human embryo is recognizably human. The brain has formed sufficiently to send out electrical impulses; even at this early stage, the brain is the co-ordinator of the other organs.

Growth is very rapid. The embryo grows at the rate of about a millimetre a day. This is not a regular growth, but the development of first one portion and then another of what will be the human body. The skeleton begins to develop when the embryo is about forty-six to forty-eight days old.

The foetus can move and be quite active during the third

---

endanger his life. In the absence of modern medicine, such incompatibilities of blood attributes led to the death of the foetus and its abortion. Today, however, it is possible to some degree to reduce the antibody formation in the blood of the mother, and even to replace the baby's blood with a transfusion of blood free from antibodies. Though some of these children are nevertheless born dead, many today can survive so that some couples who would not have been able, in the past, to bear living children with one another (though both are fertile) can become parents. Many couples, before marriage, have blood examinations made to determine whether they will encounter such difficulties. If it is discovered that they will encounter them, they can prepare for them, medically and psychologically, decide to have no children, or even decide not to marry.

month, and certainly so from that time on. It can move its limbs and soon learns to grasp. The muscular contractions which will ultimately become facial expressions can be recorded. In most cases, the mother does not feel the movement of her child until he has grown sufficiently that the uterus has expanded above the natural container formed by the pelvis, usually during the fourth or fifth month.

Obviously, the child has muscles if he moves at this early age. His nervous system is also developing – he can react to pressures and loud noises. It is believed today that the first part of the human body to become sensitive is the area of the mouth. Only later do the eyes, the hands, and other parts of the body achieve sufficient nerve endings to be sensitive to touch. By the end of the tenth week of foetal life, the only important parts of the body which are not sensitive to touch are the back and the top of the head, which will remain insensitive until after birth.

By the end of the fourth month of life, the baby has achieved half the height he will reach before birth. Certainly during the fifth month his movements can be detected by the mother. He sleeps and wakes, and has already acquired some of his favourite physical positions. During the sixth month, the child begins to acquire some fat, and also gets the buds for his permanent teeth behind the milk teeth, which are themselves developing. By the end of the sixth month the child is as much as a foot long and weighs about a pound. Fingernails have started to grow and he is very active indeed.

Pre-natal Growth and Birth

The last three months of pre-natal life see the completion of many body parts, but most of the job has been done. During this final pre-natal period the child is primarily growing, gaining weight, and achieving muscular control. By the time he is ready to be born, he is so big that his movements are extremely hampered by the restricted area now provided by the uterus. His demands are also such that the placenta is no longer able to fulfill them all.

Figure 4. The Child in utero

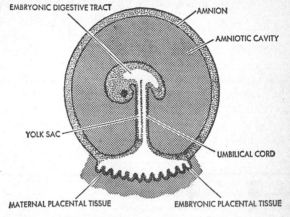

EMBRYONIC DIGESTIVE TRACT
AMNION
AMNIOTIC CAVITY
YOLK SAC
UMBILICAL CORD
MATERNAL PLACENTAL TISSUE
EMBRYONIC PLACENTAL TISSUE

A. A diagrammatic rendering of the embryo in an early stage of its development.

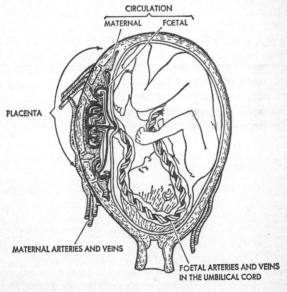

CIRCULATION
MATERNAL FOETAL
PLACENTA
MATERNAL ARTERIES AND VEINS
FOETAL ARTERIES AND VEINS IN THE UMBILICAL CORD

B. The almost fully developed foetus.

Birth begins when, as part of the normal ageing process of the placenta and the growth of the child, the placenta becomes inadequate to its task. A birth hormone (pitocin) is secreted by the pituitary. The amniotic sac breaks, releasing the fluid that has been the child's environment. The head of the child (occasionally the buttocks) presses against the cervix, beginning the muscular movements of the uterus, known as 'labour'. It is a combination of hormonal balance and this pressure that creates the contraction of the uterus. The cervix must enlarge to accommodate the baby's head, and the muscles in the uterus apply a considerable pressure. The head of the child emerges through the cervix and the enlarged vagina. The next stage requires even more force from the muscles of the uterus, for the birth to be completed. The word 'labour' is to be taken literally.

When the child is outside the mother, the umbilical cord is cut and bound; blood of course now stops flowing through it and within a week or ten days it dries and drops off.

Birth is always difficult for the baby; the bones of his head have sometimes been squeezed out of shape and there is no doubt that the process is a traumatic one. There is also a change from a liquid environment to an air environment, and there is a vast temperature difference for the baby. Breathing must begin – it is difficult at first, for the air sacs of the lungs have never before been in contact with air.

Birth takes from an hour to as many as thirty-six or even more hours, but most first births take from thirteen to sixteen hours, and most subsequent births from six to eight hours. Most babies are born tired from the struggle, but soon regain strength and normal shape.

A few people are born by surgery rather than by the normal birth processes. This operation, through the side walls of the mother's abdomen, is called 'Caesarean section', and is performed when there are physiological or medical reasons why the mother should not undergo the processes of childbirth. Babies born by Caesarean section are perfectly normal, but because the hormonal balances are not the 'triggering' mechanisms, particular care must be taken with them to see that breathing and other life processes are fully and properly established. Most doctors recommend Caesarean section only in cases of real danger to child and mother.

Abortion and Miscarriage

The death of an individual may occur before birth as well as after birth, and it is usually for the same reasons – either gross malfunction of some of the organs of the body, or disease. There are several words to be familiar with. If the pregnancy is ended, the foetus is 'aborted' if this happens before the twenty-eighth week of the pregnancy. If the foetus is aborted before the end of the twentieth week, it is called a miscarriage in some circles. The word 'abortion' is often used in the popular language to mean only artificially induced abortion. In American society, artificially induced abortion is illegal except in cases where the natural progress of pregnancy and birth would endanger the mother's life. As these lines are being written, several states, notably Colorado and California, have rewritten their laws so that legal abortion is allowable if the mother's health, either physical or mental, is in danger. Other states are studying their abortion laws, and further changes are to be expected.

Other countries – notably Denmark and Japan – have more liberal abortion.

Artificially induced abortion is not usually dangerous to the mother IF IT IS DONE BY A DOCTOR IN A HOSPITAL. However, if it is done illegally in the secrecy and in the inadequately equipped or sterilized places in which many illegal abortions are done, it may be extremely dangerous and may result in the death or permanent mutilation of the woman. There are no methods for self-induced abortion that are not even worse than those of the worst 'abortion mill'. Even to try is to court death.

Sometimes after six months of pregnancy, and certainly after seven months, babies may be born 'prematurely' and survive. They have more difficulties than do 'full-term babies' in digestive and breathing processes, but they usually survive if they are treated under hospital or equally good conditions.

From Conception to Birth

From birth until he acquires his entire full growth, the human being increases in weight an average of about twenty times. Obviously, this average covers a wide ground because the differences in weight of mature individuals are far greater than those of newly born infants. However, the difference between weight at birth and at full growth is negligible beside this astonishing figure: between conception and birth, the human creature increases in weight about SIX BILLION times.

No other change in the human condition – from the beginning to the end of life – is so great as that of birth. It thrusts the human being out of a liquid environment and into an air environment. It changes his source of nourishment from the placenta and ultimately his mother to a dependence on his own organic functions. Most important of all, perhaps, it turns him into a social creature.

Chapter 9

Post-natal Growth

The human being is born at an earlier stage of his physical development than is any other mammal (except, of course, the marsupials). Human children at birth are more dependent on the other creatures in their new external environment than are almost any other animals.

This fact goes with another – human beings have developed the art of learning to a higher degree than have any other animals. All animals, probably including the amoeba, learn a little from experience, but human beings have learned more from experience than has any other creature, and as a result more of their behaviour is dependent on learning. Indeed, the head of the human being – which, of course, contains the brain – is so large at the time of birth that were he to live an intra-uterine life any longer, he could not be born through the human birth canal as it has now evolved. Although all newborn mammals need assistance, the human baby is more nearly helpless and needs a proportionately longer part of his life to get his full growth than does any other mammal.

The Three Kinds of Needs

In short, when a baby is born he is a bundle of needs, and these needs must be satisfied. The psychiatrist Harry Stack Sullivan has divided the needs of the human infant (and, indeed, of all human beings) into three main groups. The first of these is the need for the chemicals and the proper temperature to maintain life and growth. The infant, as any other human being, feels these needs as the tensions of hunger and cold, and as the need for oxygen.

The second type of need is that for sleep. This need is one that we do not yet understand totally, although our present scientific knowledge of sleep is more extensive than it was even a few years ago. This is a difficult subject, and I shall say no more about the need for sleep than that it includes a need to dream, that the proportion of time one spends sleeping is reduced as one grows older, and that the way in which people sleep is greatly affected by their cultural customs.

The third kind of need has been called many things, but there is no real need for a euphemism – it is the need for love. This need is a response to a kind of tension quite different from the tensions of chemical demands. It is what doctors call the tension of anxiety. The tension of anxiety does not pertain to physical needs, but to the fear of punitive social relationships or of the loss of gratifying relationships.

The personality of the human animal is rooted as deeply in this need for love – at least, personal interaction – as his physical well-being is rooted in his chemical needs. The baby can no more continue to live without attention and love than he can live without food and warmth. The statement is not a metaphor – babies die without love. They can make do – survive – with terribly little. But for them to develop to the best advantage to themselves and society, only a steady and large supply will do.

The Needs of an Infant

We have already seen that birth is, from one point of view, a process which turns the biological relationship between mother and child into a social relationship. However, it is not as abrupt a change as one might think, because the chemical needs of the child are for some months, or in some societies even for two or three years, still supplied directly from the mother's breasts.

The same series of changes in the balance of the hormones of the mother which cause labour to begin and birth to proceed also trigger changes which start the flow of milk in her breasts. The first day or two after the birth, the milk is preceded by a watery fluid called colostrum, containing many hormones and other chemicals which the baby's system can utilize in its adaptation to complete dependence on its own organic system.

In the modern Western world, not all babies are suckled at their mothers' breasts. Many are fed from a bottle with a rubber nipple, containing a formula, usually made with cow's milk, occasionally with goat's milk, changed by the addition of water, glucose, and sometimes other chemicals to resemble human milk. There is a great deal of opinion, but comparatively little fact, about whether there are any differences in the growth and health of babies that are suckled at the breast and those suckled with a bottle.

It has been claimed in the past that because the mother also physically experiences nursing, it is preferable. When comparing breast feeding and bottle feeding, one should remember that suckling involves not just nourishment, but also love. It is in suckling that the child gets both. If he gets both from a breast, that is fine. If he gets both from a bottle held by his mother or some other genial and relaxed person, that is fine too (although we do not know for sure whether there are components of human milk that may be absent from formulas). The main point is, however, that the child be both nourished and loved. Unfortunately, it is possible either to nurse a child or to give it a bottle with positive dislike instead of with relaxation and love.

The tone of social life is set by the experiences of early infancy in much the same way as the tone of physical life is set by the pre-natal environment. A baby's first social relationship is with his mother – either his natural mother or an adopted mother. If the mother is a woman of perception and love and if she is not worried about something else, both of them will enjoy it.

The child experiences the relationship with his whole body, but primarily with his mouth. The mouth was the first part of the foetus to become sensitive to touch; now it is the first part of his body he must learn to control. His mouth and nose are important in breathing, and as we have already seen, the establishment of the child's own breathing is one of the critical points in human life. He must also learn to use his mouth to take in food. Some babies have been sucking their thumbs for some time before they were born. Most of the others quickly learn to suck.

Finally, the baby uses his mouth to yell – a communication that he is hungry or cold or soiled or needs some other sort of attention – including interpersonal security and love.

Indeed, the mouth is one of the most important parts of the body. From birth to death we take in through it the nourishment that keeps us alive. Through it, as tiny babies, we took in whatever fundamental emotional knowledge we have of how to love. And through it goes language – by far the most important of all our social intercommunications. The mouth is one of our primary 'social organs'.

The Needs and Accomplishments of a Child

Childhood is a time when our bodies grow and develop. With each change and growth, we experience new sensations, discover new capabilities and must learn the social limitations that are put on our capabilities. When a child is a few months old, he learns to crawl; when he is a year or so old, he begins to walk. The joy of being able to move independently and for yourself can surely be paralleled by few other physical conquests of the self and the environment. However, at that time the baby also has to begin to learn that there are ranges within which he must stay, that there are certain areas of the household or the yard that he must not wander away from. He must learn that there are many dangerous things in the world; he has to control or avoid them.

Every time a child acquires a new physical capacity, he has necessarily to learn to regulate it. He has to be taught to use his new skill within the range permitted by his family and his society. Joy must be tempered to fit the social needs. It starts with feeding, and goes on to turning over, to crawling, to walking.

Sometime soon – and the time varies with different cultures and different societies and indeed, at different historical periods in our own society – the child must learn two sets of techniques that increase his independence and self-reliance. He must learn to feed himself, and he must learn to control his bladder and his bowels.

Weaning is no longer a necessarily traumatic experience, because we have learned to prepare what we rather carelessly call 'solid' foods in such a way that they can be digested by the baby from the age of two or three weeks. Even breast-fed babies in our culture get accustomed to drinking water and orange juice from a bottle. There is thus no abrupt change from breast feeding to 'solid' food, as there is in many of the world's cultures.

Toilet training is still somewhat more difficult. Almost all animals, including birds, have ways of keeping their nests more or less clean. The young must be taught early, if they do not know it from some sort of chemical instinct, how to avoid fouling the nest. Among human beings (and probably among all other animals) toilet training demands great strength of the child, and considerable technique and control. It is possible to 'condition' even a very young baby to control his bladder and anal sphincter until certain 'triggering' situations (such as a cold toilet seat) are present. This practice is not the same thing as toilet training and most doctors advise against it. True toilet training means that the child knows when he should or should not urinate or defecate and can control his sphincters and choose where and when he will do it. The latter techniques may not be fully mastered until the age of three or four or even five.

It is important to realize that in learning mastery of his body the child is at the same time learning about the values and attitudes that his family, particularly his mother, communicates to him regarding these various bodily functions. He is learning not only about himself as an animal, but about himself as a social being.

One of the most important changes that comes about in a child is the establishment of the dominance of one side or the other of his brain. After this he is more or less unequivocally right-handed or left-handed. One side of the brain is larger, and it would seem that this growth allows for the kind of directional seeing that is necessary in order for the child to read easily. This brain dominance is established sometime between the fourth and the sixth year. It is usually established earlier in girls than boys.

With it, the child can learn to read if he is given the right kind of instruction. Some children can learn some techniques of reading and writing before brain dominance is established. We know as yet very little about the development of the brain and the way in which the co-ordination of the senses takes place as one progresses through life.

As the child approaches the age of four or five years, he becomes less immediately dependent on his mother. He does not, however, become less dependent on people – he branches out to the society of his family, his peer group, and his neighbours. The number of people on whom he depends increases. He begins to outgrow what might be called the 'general purpose relationship' with the mother, and to take on many 'special purpose relationships' with other members of the family, with friends and peers, and with teachers.

This new freedom demands that children must learn the basic social techniques of getting along with others – not only with their mothers, but also with other persons with whom they must share their mothers' attention – with the father and the siblings – and finally with people who do not even know the mother. A child must, in short, learn that to get the fullest social and physical rewards, he must sometimes forego the immediate satisfaction of needs. He must learn to postpone, for at least short periods of time, the release of tensions. Everybody must live with anxiety from time to time.

After he is about six years old, the child enters a period which the psychoanalysts call 'latency'. This rather arbitrary word means that during this period, the time of what they call 'infant sexuality' is over and the time of adult sexuality has not yet begun. During that period, which lasts from six to as many as eight years, the child is growing and learning muscular techniques – but there is no precipitous capacity such as the ability to walk or the maturation of the genitals which thrusts him into new environmental relationships. The small and delicate muscles of the hands and fingers develop during the early part of this period so that by the time he is seven or eight years old, he is capable of extremely delicate movements of his hands. Such

86

fine movements as writing, stringing beads, and the tiny movements necessary to play musical instruments or to run industrial machinery can all be learned by latency-age children. As latency proceeds, the child perfects the co-ordination of eye and hand necessary for writing or for shooting a bow and arrow or for the creation and maintenance of complex technology. He also learns to learn, as an overt technique.

Puberty

Although the growth and development of the human body is probably not complete until the age of about twenty-seven, the last major changes to be accompanied by changes in the inner sensations of experiencing the body come at the time of adolescence, or puberty. It is at this time that one becomes a fully mature creature sexually, capable of begetting or bearing children.

The development of new capacities – the muscles that allow one to walk, or to control one's bladder, or to co-ordinate the eye and the hand so that one can write – creates new responsibilities at the same time. So it is with puberty as well. At puberty the genitals grow and develop, and one acquires the physical capacity to engage in effective sexual relations and to become a parent. With this development of the body comes the necessity for a new social responsibility. One must, in short, learn to be a fully sexed and sexual being within the range of expression allowed and encouraged in one's society. We shall have more to say about this in the coming chapters of this book. Here we are interested primarily in the physiology of puberty.

Puberty is a process of growth which takes several months, or as much as a year or more, but which nevertheless seems subjectively to the person undergoing it, and to his family and friends, to be a very sudden occurrence. In girls the first sign of approaching puberty is usually the development of the breasts, although the appearance of pubic hair and of hair under the arms may precede rather than follow the development of the breasts. The first menstruation is the point at which most of the people of the world compute female puberty. In boys, puberty is usually heralded by the growth of pubic hair and the changing of the voice. It occurs between the ages of twelve and fourteen, although some boys do not reach puberty until fifteen or sixteen, and some few may achieve it as early as ten or eleven. Puberty in males is marked by growth of the genitals and emission of semen.

In primitive societies both the first emission in boys and the first menstruation in girls may be surrounded by many rituals and magical beliefs. In the past, some young people in our own society came to these experiences without the knowledge of what they are. Even today, some are frightened by them or think their parents will be distressed or angry. It is best if both boys and girls can talk to their parents about the events that are going on in their bodies at the time of puberty, for they must be made aware of what these processes are, that they are normal, not harmful, and are the sign of approaching physical and social adulthood.

After the genitals and the secondary sex characteristics – the beard, the voice, the breasts – have developed, there is a greater difference in the way the two sexes experience the world than ever before. Grown men move more rapidly than do most women. The weight on male bodies is distributed differently than on female bodies. Stronger and broader shoulders make their experiences of reaching and balancing a little different from those of women. The experience of a male body – its musculature, posture, genitals – sets and enlarges the horizons of the world as experienced by males. It is in the nature of the male genitals to quest and pierce, and it is in the nature of the human male to be thrust outward into the world that he has in one way or another to conquer. The human male is sexually aroused much more quickly than is the female, and men have a tendency to be impatient, dominant – not to say domineering – and adventurous.

Similarly, the female inhabits a chemical and sensual world different from that of the male. She has a more or less constant concern with the menstrual cycle. Her physiology makes her slower in sexual arousal, but capable of greater number of releasing orgasms. Her genitals are largely inside, and therefore do not 'get in the way' during her activities; and she experiences sexual intercourse and reproduction as something inside herself. The enfolding quality is one of the most notable qualities of the well-adjusted female personality.

Girls sometimes have another problem at puberty – when men suddenly include them in their 'girl-watching', some girls experience being a 'thing' instead of a person. One woman, trying to explain this point to me, wrote,

> It is bad enough that your body has betrayed you – instead of having something you can run and fight with, you have something that bleeds and bulges. It may take years, but it all seems very sudden. And it is made worse when boys who had not seen you or who had found you a nuisance now stare at you, and your parents' friends who never saw you before suddenly start to ogle. They all want this body you are living in. Girls who think that this is what life is all about may consider it natural that men should 'love' them, but a girl who is brought up to think of herself as an individual, maybe with brains, who happens to be female – well, it takes some getting used to.

Of course, culturally determined values and principles can reduce or expand the way either sex perceives the real world. Some activities or feelings assigned to one sex in a society might be allotted to the other sex in a different society. Neither society is 'wrong'; they have different cultures. But, once culture has been acknowledged, the fact remains – you are either a man or a woman. The greatest of all mysteries is what it would be like to be of the other sex.

Some six or seven years after puberty, the individual is ready to take up his place as a fully fledged member of society. Those six or seven years are, among the most difficult of all years of your life. The difficulty arises from the same sources as our greatest cultural accomplishments.

The development of Western culture has made it necessary for education to be prolonged beyond the primary growth processes. Whereas formerly your physical equipment was maturing and you were learning to master it, now the cultural equipment continues to accumulate and you must learn to master it. You have to learn to drive a car – which takes judgement beyond that of a child. You have to learn the principles of citizenship and the rights and obligations in an involved political world. You have to learn ways of making a living, and the almost countless techniques that are required just to run a modern n home. We all have to learn to be informed. Today, lots of us must learn the intricacies of computers, of submarines, of the human mind itself. And we must learn to make decisions – decisions about our careers, about our sex lives and our marriages, and about our ideas about justice and conflict and aggression and peace.

Because we have so much choice and so many options, we also have many problems. One of the most intense is the 'artificial' prolongation of the status of 'teenager' between the ages of puberty and the age of full-status membership in society. Necessarily, the solution to a problem of this sort rests primarily with the people who are most intimately acquainted with it – those who are living it. Older people should try, without being harsh, to understand their struggles and to assist them in finding new solutions, not merely castigate them for abandoning old ones. From the standpoint of the adolescent, this problem is one of how to be true to one's self and to develop one's self, at the same time that one is not destructive of society and culture.

Social growth has to accompany physical bodily growth. With the growth of your body and the acquisition of new knowledge and new techniques, you acquire social responsibilities. Today the demands for social and cultural growth are such that they require more time than does the maturation of the body. This is a social problem for modern technological societies that requires daring new solutions in education and in social traditions – including sexual traditions.

Part Two

The Human Dilemma

Chapter 10

Sex and Love

There is a folk tale among a people called the Tiv of central Nigeria that long ago, every man carried his wife's vagina around with him in his shoulder bag, along with his pipe and tobacco, the magical charms to protect him from witches, and whatever else constituted his daily needs. Then one day a very careless young man left his shoulder bag too close to the fire while he was busy at the smithy repairing a hoe. His wife's vagina became badly scorched. When he returned home, his wife was so angry with him that she took her vagina away from him. She organized all the women of the world, and they agreed that all of them would keep their vaginas with them always. And ever since that time, every vagina has been permanently attached to a woman.

The point of this Tiv tale is that all sexual relationships involve people with personalities, and that a sexual relationship is an intimate form of social relationship that goes far beyond the sex act. We in our culture make this point by asking a searching question: 'Is what I feel love or is it "just sex"?' 'How can you tell the difference?'

It is one of the greatest achievements of Western civilization that it has succeeded in culturally linking the physical drive of sexuality with the emotion of love, which Westerners today consider the most 'noble' of emotions. This linking is not 'natural'. It is, rather, a cultural discovery.

A difficulty arises when we Westerners are taught to think that there is a natural and 'normal' association between sex and love, when in fact this association is a cultural value. Since it is a cultural value, we must learn it just as we must learn any other cultural values. The question 'Is what I feel sex or love?' must be interpreted as a request for more information about the way in which the physical drive and the emotion are to be hooked together.

Sex and the Emotions

Sexual activities are a source of considerable emotion in human beings. The reason is not merely the excitement of sexual arousal – it is just as importantly the ethical and cultural considerations that unavoidably accompany it.

Sex is not an emotion. It is one of the animal drives. Emotions are the ways we are taught to feel about our drives: a quality in the way we experience our drives. A drive can be suppressed for longer or shorter periods of time, or it can be displaced from its area of origin to some other area of physical or social living. But a drive remains, fundamentally, a raw quantity of energy. Emotions, on the other hand, are qualities that we learn to assign to the drives and to the ways we express them. Emotions are tied up with our attitudes about other people and with our images of the self. Emotions are 'educated' ways of perceiving and thinking and feeling about not only our drives, but about other people and about morality.

All human beings have, to one degree or another, surrounded sexuality with emotion and a set of ideals. A few peoples of the world have associated sexuality with evil and darkness; a few others have tried to make it a religious exercise. But wherever it may be, the community in which a person lives always prescribes and to some degree controls the emotions that it considers suitable or allowable in sexual matters.

It is possible to use sexuality as a weapon and to copulate in anger; in a few places in the primitive world, mass rape is a recognized mode of punishment. It is possible to link sexuality with emotions such as shame or even fear. Many religions have linked sexuality with spiritual visions. It is even possible, to a degree at least, to de-emotionalize it so that one copulates in what appears to be a state of non-commitment or disinterest.

Therefore, information about our mammalian biology – and the drives that are a part of it – is not enough to guide or inform our conduct, although it is the necessary place to start. Of equal importance with biology is what people are taught to think about their bodies, about their drives, and about their acts.

Every human being must experience and explore his body. He unavoidably has emotions about it: he may consider it beautiful and strong and good, or he may consider it ugly and evil. These emotions are learned responses, most of them unconsciously learned. Every human being must experience the drives within him – this is the perception of the chemical workings of his living organism, and he necessarily feels these chemical reactions with his attitudes intact – either that his drives are the source of his power and love, or that they are shameful.

Every human being acts. And he evaluates his acts in accordance with the reactions of the other people in his community. Doing nothing can, of course, be a significant act.

You need not act on your feelings. That does not mean that you have to deny to yourself that you feel them. To admit to yourself that you would like to have a sexual adventure with somebody you know does not, obviously, mean that you have to rush out and do it. To refuse to act on your feelings is often a form of social competence – just as acting in accordance with your feelings, when the situation is 'right', is also a form of social competence. But to deny that you have feelings is an act of self-delusion, ultimately even of self-destruction. Feelings, both drives and emotions, can be judged by others only if you act on them or tell somebody what they are. Acts can be destructive of other people. Emotions hidden from the self can be self-destructive. The only sensible way out of the dilemma is to admit the emotions to one's self, then act in the best interests both of the self and of other people. This may mean that acts are repressed – but not that the emotions are repressed.

There are, thus, two sets of questions: 'What am I allowed to do? What do I do?' And, then, on the other hand, 'What do I feel?'

Both sets of questions should be answered with knowledge and with honesty. But before we know what we feel and what we can do, we have to recognize the evaluative lens through which we are observing the biological facts and the emotional facts.

Love: The Adventure in Intimacy

Love is a complex emotion because it involves both the self and others outside the self. Therefore it is always an aspect of a relationship ('secret love' is not love, although all love cannot be fulfilled). Like 'life' in general, love embodies what appears to be a contradiction: the satisfaction of the self through the satisfaction of the needs and desires of others.

Far from being selfless, love provides a double satisfaction – even a triple satisfaction – to the self: once to the self because you can love and are loving; once to the self when love is reciprocated and you are loved; and once to the self because you know that, since you are loving and being loved, you must have a lovable self. When it is all there, you are well and truly 'locked in'. Nobody wants out.

Love, being an emotion, does not spring up full-blown with sexual maturity. If a person is lucky, he has learned to love in a long process that begins within a few hours of birth.

However, at puberty, love must be brought into focus with the sexual drive. Love of parents, brothers and sisters, and friends continues. But love is now also associated with the sex drive and turns you to courtship, perhaps love affairs, probably eventual marriage.

There are many different aspects to a relationship of love between a man and a woman. Here I shall consider only four of them. The fact that they are the four which lead into marriage is not empty moralizing on my part: it is, rather, a fact of Western culture. Every courtship between a man and a woman, whether it is sexually consummated or not, and whether it leads to marriage or not, starts down this track. It is easy to throw the relationship off the track, to break it at any point – including after marriage, as we shall see.

The four aspects of love that I want to discuss are:

1. Companionship,
2. Sexuality,
3. Domesticity,
4. Co-parenthood.

In accordance with the values of our society, these four aspects of love are increasingly associated with marriage. None of them has to be associated with marriage, although if they are not, more social difficulties appear with each added element. Many societies do not have any overt concepts about 'love' as we have, yet these four aspects are to be found in most places, in some degree and in some mixture.

Depending on the nature of the society and culture at hand, these different aspects of love can be differentially explored by the unmarried. Our own society is very permissive about companionship, much less permissive about sex, it condemns householding among the unmarried (although a lot of it is to be found), and it condemns unmarried co-parenthood out of hand (although the illegitimacy rates in America and Europe are not low ones).

Companionship. Americans and Europeans think that the companionship side of the love relationship 'should' be explored before marriage. Companionship is an element in all friendship as well as in heterosexual love. The intimacy of companionship begins to be built up when you reveal yourself to the other and, in most cases (else the relationship would cease), realize that what you have revealed is approved or even cherished by the other person. That in itself is vastly gratifying. Then, in response, you are shown more of the personality of the other, and if you can approve, you do. In almost a rapture of discovery further revelations and acceptances occur. That is friendship. It is also Western love at the 'introductory level'.

Sex and Love. If what you are feeling is love and not 'just sex', the companionship and friendship precede the sexualizing of the relationship. I am not knocking 'just sex'. I am saying that if a relationship begins with sex, it is apt to end there. It may run into what might be called the '*second*-hour syndrome'. No one

97

should ever begin an affair without asking, 'What could we do the second hour?' If the second hour can be filled with friendship, then you may be on the road to love. If it cannot, that is a sure sign (one of many) that it is 'just sex'.

Sexuality, without doubt, deepens a relationship. But if the relationship cannot be happily sustained after or without sex, then something is wrong somewhere: either in the emotional capacity of the people to want to get involved or stay involved, or merely in their personal incompatibility. A relationship cannot survive on the strength of sex alone.

People in some societies are allowed to explore some aspects of sexuality before marriage. They cannot explore them all, simply because the people of the community treat them differently before and after marriage. Our own society theoretically does not 'allow' premarital sex but often tacitly permits some relationships if they are inconspicuous. (The affairs of movie stars and other notables are usually intended to be flagrant.)

In the middle classes, the attitude of most people towards sexual intercourse of couples who are 'properly engaged' is more lenient than to couples who are not engaged – and some couples even use an 'engagement' (which can, after all, be broken fairly easily) as a ruse or an excuse.

Domestic and Co-Parental Aspects. When it comes to the domestic and co-parental aspects of love and intimacy, even less can be learned before marriage – especially by those who are making their first experiments with householding. A more rigid rule of etiquette always applies before marriage than after – and greater intimacy is achieved after it. There is always an assumption that the same standards will apply after the marriage as did before – but it is not always so. I know a Frenchman who married his mistress of twenty-five years – an impeccable housekeeper. She took to her bed two weeks after the marriage and never again did cooking or cleaning. Educated and shrewd guesses are possible – and some people may have been right enough in their guesses that they will challenge my statement. They are fortunate.

Then, finally, comes the couple's adjustment to being coparents. Obviously, many couples encompass this experience with a minimum of difficulty and a maximum of reward, because love has proved itself and found new fields to explore and enjoy. Just as obviously, however, many others go through a bad period and some of them come to grief. It is never possible to 'know' what kind of parent your spouse is going to be. A flamboyant dancer, a fine lover, an ample provider or neat housekeeper – none is a guaranteed good parent.

Of course, it is possible to make guesses about parent potential on the basis of the background and home life of the other person. It is possible to watch him with children. But it is not possible to know the covert assumptions that the other person has about the nature of parenthood or even adulthood. Until put to the test, there is probably little opportunity for these unspoken assumptions to come to the surface.

Something even more subtle is also at work: it is impossible before marriage really to know yourself as a domestic person. There is really no way to know what kind of a parent you yourself will make. Therefore, you are not just *marrying* an unknown; you yourself are an unknown. Yet, most people do, with good reason, trust their inner natures.

This oversimplified pattern of love extends through time. It begins in companionship and grows to include co-parenthood. It is necessary, in the Western world, to assume that love leads to marriage if it is to reach completeness.

At the time of most marriages, the parties know that they are satisfactory companions, and many of them today know that they are at least potentially satisfactory sexual partners. They know comparatively little about the domestic talents and requirements of one another, and they know next to nothing about the qualities they will exhibit as parents.

Breaking Off an Intimate Relationship

An intimate relationship may be arrested any place along its line of progress. Ultimately, as we shall see in the chapter on marriage, it *must* be arrested if the personalities are not to be swamped and if the two selves are to retain or gain auto-nomy, which (ironically) is necessary for a love relationship to deepen.

Arresting such a relationship is not the same thing as breaking it off. Many relationships 'go too far', and therefore the people feel that they must break them off rather than try to backtrack to make them less intense. No person is ever quite the same again after a relationship of real intimacy – his self has been bent towards that other person. Men forget call girls – but they do not forget intimate friends or the women they have loved. Women may forget 'one-night stands' – but if they have loved and been loved they do not forget, and their characters have been per-manently affected.

Many people choose, more or less consciously, not to let any particular relationship, or perhaps any relationship at all, 'go too far'. All this is a personal matter, which can be more or less controlled by the individual, especially in the absence of that parasite on love called romantic love.

Romantic Love

Romantic love is a situation that occurs when one's love fanta-sies become ends in themselves – when one is seeking love as one seeks medicine for an ailment. Historical research into the origins of romantic love among the fourteenth-century trouba-dours of Catalonia and southern France has brought to light fascinating moralities: it allows us to understand medieval litera-ture and much about medieval society. However, a shift in the meaning of the term 'romantic love' confused the present-day meaning of the historical ideas. Whatever its origins, middle-class love today has very little indeed to do with the romantic love of the troubadours.

Romantic love, as it occurs today, is a sort of psychological love potion that some people either administer to themselves or else use as an excuse when they want to be irresponsible.

The explanation of its use is simple: in the explorations of in-timacy, 'romantic love' enters any time you are unable or unwilling to face the facts and see what is there. Instead, the need for affection, the sexual urges, histrionic self-display, or just plain loneliness – any or all of them may make it desirable for a person to blind himself to the real nature of the other person's personality and his own. This state is sometimes called 'falling in love with love'. That kind of love *is* blind – it has been blinded so that you will not have to give it up when you see the disadvantages for you in the personality of the 'loved one'. If you need the advantages enough, the disadvantages may momentarily even seem a small price to pay, so you discard awareness of them. Love affairs founded on this kind of self-deception are unfortunate. Marriages founded on such self-deception may be tragic.

Therefore, it is vital to make a distinction between love and romantic love. Love sees clearly – it may accept faults, but it does not blind itself to them. Romantic love is blind – wilfully blind, because it will not look. Romantic love is a form of enchantment; love is a clear way of looking at the real world.

Many cultures of the world fail to distinguish sufficiently between love and romantic love. Many Americans and Europeans do not make a clear enough distinction, with the result that some love affairs and some marriages are founded on illusion. Other cultures do not make the distinction, and then logically enough claim that 'love' (by which they mean romantic love) is the worst basis for a marriage, because its presence has nothing to do with what these peoples consider to be suitable qualities in spouses. Arranged marriages, in all societies which practise the custom, result from more or less intense care given to the selection of suitable spouses so that companionship and co-parenthood can grow, leading to love.

Westerners find themselves in the position of *saying* that nothing matters for marriage except love. If they mean the genuine article, I have no quarrel with them. But sometimes they confuse real love with romantic love. Fortunately, even some people who suffer from the confusion do not practise what they preach. Through common sense and the growth of real love, qualities of good will, motherliness or manliness, intelligence, strength, and a moral upbringing may be 'bootlegged' even into the wildest-seeming 'romantic love'. But when moon and June and the biological drives lead you to blind yourself, these qualities may fail to get in at all.

Chapter 11

Sex and Non-Love

Children, in the course of their emotional development, sometimes get sex mixed up with fantasies of which they are frightened.
It was one of the greatest discoveries of Sigmund Freud that
such terrifying fantasies can be thrust out of consciousness, but
not totally forgotten. When we are adults, the unconscious but
not forgotten fantasies may affect our lives in many ways. One
of the most obvious ways is that such people must make their
sexual adjustments only in areas beyond these fantasies so that
the fantasies themselves – and the fear they aroused – can be kept
out of consciousness.

All this is the normal working of the human mind. But if the
original fear was too great, it sometimes leads to unfortunate
results. There are two basic kinds of these results, both so inter-
linked with normal processes that it is difficult to say where the
'pathology' may begin. One result is the kind of neurosis that
occurs when one of the non-love emotions becomes primary in a
person's sexual feeling. Most normal adults, on some occasions,
experience mixtures of many emotions involved with their sexual
activities. These mixtures of emotions are usually harmless, and
can be explained by the situation of the moment and by the
history of the individual through whom these emotions are cours-
ing. However, when the fantasies were suppressed to hide the
painfulness of love, the non-love emotions may be the only ones
that are available to be associated with the sexual drive.

Change of Target: Homosexuality

A second way of dealing with the unconscious fear is to change the target of the sexual urges.

We have already noted that although love and sex go together, some kinds of love are kept apart from sexuality. Attraction for – love of – members of the same sex is normal. It is to be found in everybody. Most people do not, of course, sexualize this attraction. However, if there is a block to normal sexual expression, some may. Any sexual act that takes place between people of the same sex is called homosexual. Close, intense friendships between boys or between girls are not in themselves homosexual; they do not even indicate what is sometimes called 'latent' homosexuality (which means that the homosexual impulses are either unrecognized or are under control and never indulged). Non-sexual, but nevertheless intense, friendships between persons of the same sex are especially common among adolescents, but they exist throughout life and are richly rewarding.

However, homosexual acts do occur. Most of them involve no more than mutual manual masturbation. However, mouth-genital contacts may be engaged in either by men or by women, as may anal copulation by men and a form of mutual clitoral contact by women.

Alfred Kinsey and his associates showed that a large proportion of American males, and a somewhat smaller but still large proportion of American females, have engaged in homosexual relationships at least once in their lives. With very few of them, however, did that experience lead to a lasting commitment to homosexuality. One of Kinsey's finest insights was to insist that the word 'homosexual' should be applied to acts and not to those people who commit them a few times.

The confirmed homosexual person is another matter. He or she is unable, in many cases, to engage in sexual relations with members of the opposite sex.

It is sometimes thought by uninformed laymen that homosexuality is a pathology in the body chemistry. Others would like to place the blame for it on inadequacies in biological equipment, or to consider it some sort of physical abnormality. Such is almost never the case. Biological hermaphroditism (individuals who show a mixture of male and female primary sex characteristics) or genetic intersex (where the chromosomes contain both male and female features) are rare. Most homosexuals are physically perfectly normal males or females.

Rather, the difficulty that leads to homosexuality is a psychic difficulty. It almost always arises out of the fantasies that I referred to at the beginning of this chapter: a person unconsciously gets certain horrible fantasies so closely correlated with heterosexual relationships that he must, when he grows up, either change his target or do without any sexual relationships at all. The pain and frustration are as great as if there were a physical cause – perhaps greater.

Confirmed, constant, and habitual homosexuality (unlike the occasional homosexual encounter) always arises from some difficulty in the formation of the learned capacity to love, or from inability to esteem one's self highly enough to think one is lovable. Psychiatrists can usually explain individual cases of confirmed homosexuality, and many cases can be treated and cured. There is a myth that homosexuality cannot be cured because the individual gets all his sexual rewards from it, and he is afraid that giving it up might mean he would have to forego all sexual outlets. Today, many psychiatrists claim that such an explanation is over-simple and that the condition can indeed be alleviated.

Some people are also 'bisexual' – that is, they enjoy and engage in relations with their own sex as well as with people of the other sex. Indeed, a few homosexuals marry and have families without giving up homosexuality entirely. This is a form of homosexuality which does not cancel out the heterosexual desires and abilities. Obviously, it arises from different suppressed fantasies.

We do not know how common homosexuality is. Most of the statistics about the number of homosexuals in any country are incomplete, and some are downright misleading, especially the figures issued by societies of homosexuals who are attempting to get legal and social recognition of themselves and to do away with the severe legal restrictions under which they live. Collecting information on the subject of homosexuality is always difficult.

Some states in America, and some countries such as Great Britain, have in the past legislated homosexuality into a crime. This means that persons detected may be taken to court (though the number who are is very small). The laws against homosexuality are now, gradually and quietly, being repealed or ignored when the homosexual acts take place in private between consenting adults. The law in Britain which made homosexuality a crime was repealed in the middle 1960s. There are several American states which have also repealed such laws. These laws (like those against 'fornication', meaning here sexual intercourse between persons other than married partners) were seldom enforced except in cases where specific malefactors could be arrested on this charge but not on some other for which they were actually wanted. It is something like getting Al Capone for income tax evasion, instead of for more heinous crimes.

Where such laws have not been repealed, they are under heavy attack, because they allow considerable blackmail to take place and because they encourage police interference in what many people believe to be a private sector of one's life. Many important groups such as churches and civic organizations have, without condoning homosexuality, pointed out that it is not *per se* physically harmful, that confirmed homosexuals can have satisfactory social relationships with one another, and with anyone else in all the non-sexual aspects of their lives; such statements have added that much of the difficulty has come from the fact of its illegality. A few moralities in historical and present-day societies have even claimed special virtue for homosexual relationships: ancient Greece is probably the best known.

'Public nuisance' is another matter, and will probably remain a crime, because it is done in public. 'Molestation of children' will also in all probability remain a criminal act, for most societies think children should be protected until they are old enough and experienced enough to achieve a socially approved sexual autonomy.

Change of Target: Paedophilia

Another form of perversion leads some adults to seek sexual contacts with children, of either the same or the opposite sex. Paedophilia, which is derived from the Greek meaning 'love of children', may be either heterosexual or homosexual. Some aspects of it are natural enough – all young people make models out of some of their older contemporaries, and any adult may have an emotional attachment to some of the younger people who make an ideal of him. He sees in those young people good qualities that he finds attractive and wishes to help develop. In a few cases, the adult who is unable to make sexual adjustments to other adults may pervert this attraction to sexual ends. If paedophilia is combined with difficulties for that person in associating sex with love at all, and if he associates it with rage, the result is sometimes dangerous to the lives of the children.

Paedophilia is another example of a socially unprofitable association of sex with the wrong partner. Although pre-pubertal sexual activity is usually not physically harmful, it almost always disturbs the emotional development of a child.

The cause of paedophilia, as of homosexuality, is that unconscious fantasy fears associated with sex block the adult's capacity to find or approach mature sex partners.

Children should know about the possibility of paedophilia in adults – either in strangers or in people they know well. In fact, a large majority of instances of paedophilia are performed by acquaintances or kinsmen, not by strangers. A child should know how to deal with such people: to avoid them in any except large gatherings, and, of course, to refuse to accept favours from strangers.

All adults who feel sexual attraction for children should know that their condition can almost always be alleviated with psychiatric assistance. Because people who suffer from this difficulty almost without exception wish heartily to be rid of it and to be able to approach and find adult heterosexual partners, the paedophile cooperates readily with the psychiatrist, when he knows

107

that changes can be fairly rapidly brought about in his own feelings.

Sex and the Emotions Other Than Love

There are other, more subtle, forms that the emotions of 'non-love' can take in colouring the sexual appetites. These occur when the 'target' is not changed, but when the emotional commitment is not love or healthy lust, carried out with full respect of the partner. These 'perversions' result when strong non-love emotions such as hate or revenge or thirst for power are associated with sexual activity.

Perhaps the non-love emotion most commonly associated with sex in a 'perverse' kind of way is hate. Hate is not merely the absence of love, and is rather more than the opposite of love. Hate, or something like it, is likely to emerge when a person fears that he will be or has been rejected, and that love or esteem has been denied to him or might be taken away from him. Hate sometimes leads to a great desire to 'get even', and to hurt the world before it hurts you.

Some men – often called 'Don Juans' – spend years searching for love. They seduce and fornicate with as many women as they can possibly find. But love eludes them, almost always because what they are looking for is self-esteem. Because they so fear that love will not be given them, their own hate steps in before love can possibly emerge. And they go destructively from one woman to the next.

Women who exhibit a similar syndrome, for similar reasons, are usually called 'nymphomaniacs'. They are constantly in search of a love which is unfindable either because it is unreal, or because it is too soon masked by their own hate in response to their own fear. They – like the men – may even do it in an unconscious need to 'get even' with the world or whoever in it provided the original psychic injury that has been 'forgotten'.

The act of sexual intercourse, for many such people, becomes an act of aggression. We have only to go to the slang of English to know how thoroughly the four-letter sexual terms are used to express hostility and aggression.

Sometimes the sexual drive can become associated with fear. In these cases, the result is most often the suppression, sometimes the total suppression, of sexuality – that is, impotence in men and frigidity in women. Fear must be very strong to inhibit the sexual drive completely, and such people sometimes change targets in order to get some sexual release.

Indeed, the sexual drive can sometimes be associated with an awe that is nearly religious – there is comparatively little of such association to be found in the modern West, though it was found among medieval mystics and even today one sometimes hears sexual love extolled as of the same order as divine love.

Sometimes, of course, sexuality can drive one without particular emotion: lust as an end in itself, and its satisfaction accomplished without fear, anger, awe, or love. There is no regard for the partner one way or the other: either as loved, as hated, or as conquered. For all that they are not sexually frustrated, such people miss a lot – the normal development of emotional experience.

The change in target for sex or the denial or elusiveness of love are both felt by almost all who suffer from them – even those who most aggressively deny such feelings – as severe handicaps in living. However, they need not be feared and hidden, because in today's world help is available.

Chapter 12

Masturbation

Masturbation is the technical word for the act of stimulating your own genitals, especially if you reach orgasm that way. This discussion of masturbation has been put into a separate chapter, because it most certainly is not a perversion; it also is not a relationship of love. Yet it is a universal phenomenon. One of the problems that must be dealt with by all adolescents is their attitudes toward masturbation. Obviously, masturbation is not solely an adolescent activity, but nevertheless it must be faced first at that time, and attitudes are formed at that time.

There is no physical difference, either for men or women, between orgasms achieved by masturbation and those achieved in sexual intercourse. Thus, masturbation is not – obviously, it cannot be – physically harmful. It does not cause feeble-mindedness, pimples, or hair on the palms, all of which have been, in years past, more or less seriously claimed. A great many of these weird and false stories about the physical harmfulness of masturbation were circulated when your parents and grand-parents were young, though they are less in evidence today. Some of these stories grew out of a superstition that every human male manufactured only so much semen, and when it was gone his masculinity disappeared. Scientific discovery of the processes of spermatogenesis has made nonsense of that superstition. Other stories grew out of the nineteenth century superstition that it was unnatural for females to have any sexual impulses at all.

A cynic might note that masturbation was perhaps the only thoroughly disapproved single act that was widespread enough to be common to almost all men and women, and hence the only thing they held in common sufficiently that it could possibly be considered the source of all personal fault and misfortune.

The only possible danger from masturbation is psychic. Masturbation may, by some religions, still be considered as sinful. That is a matter for religious belief. It is not physically harmful – that is a matter of scientific fact. In those communities or religious sects which consider it a sin, or in which it is severely repressed, masturbation may lead to great guilt feelings. The guilt can seriously undermine a person's esteem for himself as a full-bodied and full-fledged man or woman.

As one psychoanalyst explains it, masturbation is available as a source of consolation, pleasure, and relief of tension before it is possible to link one's sexuality with love and with a loved person. Linking up with a loved person always takes time; the linkage is always subject to periods of greater or lesser disruption. Thus masturbation is available during such times of disruption also. Another psychiatrist told me that in his practice, the most frequent disorder of masturbation was its total inhibition. However, he added that compulsive masturbation – continual and to orgasm – always indicates some sort of an anxiety that is not helped by the masturbation. Although it is a relief from sexual tensions, it is not an adequate relief from the tensions of fear and aggression. The real medical problem is to find the true source of the tension and anxiety.

Self-regard and self-esteem lie at the basis of all love. Masturbation in healthy people is no more than a relief of tension for those who have not yet found, or are separated from, the persons they love. Lack of understanding about this matter or unduly severe repression of it may lead to the kind of guilt that kills self-esteem, and with it the basis on which love can be built.

Chapter 13

Self-Esteem and 'Your Own Thing'

Love begins in a tiny baby's reaction to mothering. It begins in body chemistry as well. The nursing mother gets satisfaction from being suckled by her child. A woman usually feels this as a pleasantness through her entire body. Nursing is sometimes accompanied by slight contractions of the uterus, although her feelings are not specifically sexual in nature. Even if she uses a bottle, she gets tremendous psychic satisfaction and security from providing for her child.

The nursing child gets his food and his security, and the pleasure of being held, watched, and approved. The act of giving and getting nourishment thus becomes in itself an act of love, involving physical satisfactions.

Nursing. whether by breast or bottle, cannot be done in an emotional vacuum. It is always accompanied by an emotional tone. From a good and comforting emotional tone, the child begins to think himself worthy of love, and hence he can learn to love.

Self-Love and Self-Esteem

One of the most astonishing uses of the word 'love' occurs when we begin to think about our attitudes to ourselves. It is said to be wrong and 'narcissistic' to 'love ourselves'. In the Greek myth, Narcissus was the son of a nymph and a salacious god who had raped her. Narcissus grew up to be a magnificently handsome youth, but he had never learned to love, and he spurned everyone who was attracted to him. Finally, he saw his own reflection in a pool of water and drowned in the effort to grasp its perfection in his arms.

Narcissus is the arch-example of a man who never learned he was lovable and thus could not love. His mother, the ravaged nymph, hated his father and could not care for and love the child. Narcissus would not trust others lest they betray him and ultimately drowned because he did not dare lose sight of himself.

A more modern and less mythical way to explain narcissism is this: if a child is not loved when he is a baby, he grows up feeling himself unlovable. If he feels unlovable, he always watches for unfavourable signs in other people's attitudes towards him. Therefore he can never lose sight of superficialities of social relationships long enough to trust somebody else to love him. And, in such a state, he cannot love anybody. If a person cannot feel himself worth loving, he cannot abandon himself to the emotions of love.

'Self-love' has a nasty connotation, so we must first find some new words. 'Self-esteem' is the word that we shall give to your assurance, down deep, that you are lovable. Only with self-esteem can you truly give your love – and hence be truly loved.

'Self-love', on the other hand, is not love at all, in any definition of the word. It varies from a constant watchfulness of the self so that you will not make yourself repulsive (and hence all social relations remain superficial), to a conviction that you are hateful or so gross that you can never risk being rejected and hence never get close enough to anybody to love them or to be loved. Self-love, seen this way, is one of the most unfortunate of fates. Self-esteem, on the other hand, is the base on which all love and lovableness are built.

Ethics

Valuing the mother's generosity and sympathy, the child builds these qualities into his own character. In demonstrating them, he is respecting other people's standards and so he learns that

113

others love him and respect his standards. He learns, then, the human ethic – the basic concern of human beings for one another that allows them to live together without destroying each other and the very world in which they are living. The Golden Rule of the Bible is a basically ethical statement – indeed, *the* ethical statement: do unto others as you want them to do unto you. Kant's categorical imperative is a refinement of the same idea: act only in such a way that you would be willing to take the consequences if your act were to become the universal law. Kant said this in many different ways – perhaps the most important for our purposes is his admonition that we must always treat human beings, whether ourselves or others, as an end – never merely as a means to an end.

The Ethics of Sex

There are two simple points to an ethic of sexuality. First (1) it is unethical to allow your judgement to be clouded temporarily so that you act without heed to your real standards and to future consequences. Sexual intimacy that has no meaning beyond immediate sensual satisfaction, without regard for your partner, deprives you of the pleasure of giving in total awareness – and that is the maximum pleasure. You must understand completely the value of your action – to yourself and to others. Second (2) it is unethical to lead other people astray or seduce them, or to take advantage of their weaknesses before they have decided, ethically, what their course of action is to be. If by emotional pressure or physical force or alcohol somebody's basic ideas are overrun, and he or she is made to do something that he does not really want to do but is 'arm-twisted' into doing, then that is not pleasant, not a victory for one's self, nor very much fun. It is a perversion of the need for power rather than a means of dealing with lust.

We are all far beyond the Edwardian kind of seduction, in which the villain takes advantage of the heroine. I am talking about people who are kidding themselves – like the thousands of middle-class girls who, every year, end up in homes for unmarried mothers and then place their bastard children out for adoption. Social scientists have found that most such girls have one thing in common: they know about contraceptives, but refuse to use them. To do so would prove to themselves that they are 'bad girls'. They therefore make their boy friends seduce them. This is grossly unethical behaviour. Not only did he seduce her – she seduced him into seducing her. She was afraid or unwilling to admit what she was going to do. She was treating human beings – her lover and herself – as a means to an end – her own illicit pleasure (and I use the word 'illicit' not out of my morality, but out of hers). I am also talking about the men and women who, in moments of passion, make promises they do not intend rationally to keep, or who use serious people casually. I am talking about men who promise marriage or riches or a job – promises they do not intend to keep. I am talking about women who trap men into marrying them.

The ethics of any society must be built on respect for the autonomy of other people, within at least some of the areas of life. Indeed, the ethic of twentieth-century democracy involves such a respect for autonomy of the individual in far broader areas of life than do the ethics of some other types of society. Yet, within all, a basic regard for the rights of other people is fundamental. The ethics of sexuality is a part of more general ethics, and – let us repeat it – the basis of a good society.

Morality

Unlike ethics, morality is relative. Moralities are subject to change. They vary from one society to another, from one historical period to another, and from one segment of the present-day population to another. One of the dictionaries I consulted about this word says that morality means 'virtuous behaviour according to civilized standards of right and wrong'. The point of my argument here is that it did not say what virtue was or which civilization it had in mind – it assumed you knew that, thus making my point.

Changes in morality can be studied in literature from Petronius to *One Hundred Dollar Misunderstanding*, from George Eliot to Henry Miller, from Rabelais to Gide. It can be studied in the archives of history – from the age of Constantine to the age of Victoria; from Nero to the Marquis de Sade. Moralities can be investigated in the light of the great-man theory: St Paul, Martin Luther, Sigmund Freud – all of them (and many others) were highly ethical men who were instrumental in changing the morals of their times.

The Morals of Sexuality

The varieties of morality can also be investigated by examining a broad range of societies of the world – the method which I, being an anthropologist, prefer to follow.

In the culture of the Trobriand Islands, off the northern coast of New Guinea, sexual freedom begins when children are about five years old. Their games and activities include sex games, which the adults know about and sometimes laugh at, but do not discourage. At puberty, young people are allowed to form sexual associations, and their trysting places are usually known and avoided by the adults of the community. The boys build bachelor houses, where their girl friends visit them to spend the nights. There is a strict code of etiquette within the bachelor house, and there is a complete absence of orgiastic partying, and no switching of partners or voyeurism. Such conduct is considered immoral and is not tolerated – anyone who might begin it is excluded by the bachelors themselves. By the late teens, couples have formed who will ultimately marry. Marriage is monogamous for commoners (although the chiefs may have several wives), and is more stable than marriage in our own society. The Trobrianders, in their adventure in intimacy, are encouraged to begin with sex, and then to base their marriage preferences on comradeship. Only after marriage is it permissible for a couple to live in the same household, or even to eat together.

Such moralities are misunderstood by Westerners, who assume that if there is complete sexual freedom there is never any impetus to get married. That is never the case – when premarital sexual freedom is the norm it never, in itself, interferes with the stability of marriage. Comparatively few people in any society are willing to give up the companionship and domesticity and co-parenthood that marriage implies in exchange for mere sexual freedom, especially when the sexual capacities and attributes of the spouse are well known and appreciated. In Africa my cook once asked me for an advance on his pay so that he could make a downpayment on the bride-price for a wife. He had selected one of the local girls, whom everybody (including me) thought a beauty and a healthy hard worker. I asked him why he wanted to get married. He replied that he was tired of begetting other men's children and wanted some of his own. I advanced him the money.

Many people also assume that a 'sexual revolution' is a social revolution. It is not. The family is and will remain the modular unit in American society as in every other human society (though some persons in all societies reject families). Premarital sexual freedom, where it is condoned, does not lead to new family patterns; indeed, it may lead to better social control of the actions of young people than does a policy of condemning and then winking.

Among the Tiv of Nigeria, whom I studied for almost three years, there is a traditional institution (now largely fallen into disuse because of missionary objection) in which a young couple, when he is thirteen or fourteen and she is a few years younger, are allowed to form an institutionalized sexual union. The two must be distantly related to one another (though they must not share a common grandparent, for then their sexual relations would be considered incestuous), and the parents of both are concerned parties to the arrangement. The boy is allowed to come to the hut of the girl's mother and sleep with the girl there any time the young people decide, and for as long as they care to continue. A girl seldom has more than one such lover (and never more than one at a time), and these unions last up to two or three years, before the girl gets married. If she becomes pregnant – and most do not – she is married to someone else, who becomes the social father of her child. Such a pregnancy is not a bar to marriage among the Tiv – indeed, it has proved that the girl is fertile. When I inquired about the moral reasoning behind this custom, the mother of one such girl told me, 'This way, the adults are in control – we know who is sleeping with whom, and where they are. It is better than having them off roaming around the countryside.'

At the other extreme are the Koryak of Siberia. In the early nineteenth century, before they became Russianized, they did not allow any kind of association at all between boys and girls. Sexual intercourse before marriage was a capital crime. And examples are given from the memories of old people in which guilty lovers were in fact executed. In Spain during the Middle Ages, it was incumbent on the brothers of a girl who had 'lost her honour' to kill her and also to kill her lover: the brothers' honour was stained by the same sexual act by which she had lost hers. There are even records in which brothers have been executed when they took personal revenge by castrating their sister's lover rather than society's toll by killing him.

Modern Americans and Europeans fall someplace in between these extremes. We say that sex before marriage should not be permitted. We also have a high illegitimate birth rate and a brisk sale of contraceptives to the unmarried. Obviously there is something of a gap between what we say we should do and what we in fact do.

Either to sigh and pine that our morality is changing, or to become an activist demonstrator for a 'new morality' is to be a social actor, but not to understand what is happening. Morality has *always* been changing – somebody has always been sighing and dragging his feet, and somebody else has always been demonstrating. To see it is so, you need only enlarge your time span a little.

The ideals or goals of behaviour are, in every society, set higher and made more restrictive than some people can or will follow. Young people have to realize that it is not hypocritical for a society to maintain stricter standards than some people can meet. Their parents' generation has to realize that it is not hypocritical or dangerous to explain that there are rules for making sure that when some people compromise the principles, they do not compromise them too far.

Every community has rules about who may copulate with whom. Every community also has to deal with impulse and so must have rules for those breaking the rules. In every society there are canons of morality about the conditions in which sex is allowed: admonitions about what boundaries must not be transgressed, and what punishments will be meted out to those who 'go too far'. But there is also, everywhere, a more or less hidden proposition about the conditions under which the punishments will be mitigated or suspended.

There is probably no society in which the hypocrisy has been greater than in our own about the rules for breaking the rules of sexual conduct. We have made very heavy going of the ethics and morality by which we teach young people to live and (occasionally) to compromise.

In order to understand the regulations of sexual behaviour – or of any other kind of social behaviour – it is wise to distinguish two different sets of admonitions. There are ethical rules underlying the workings of every society; they change comparatively little from one age to the next or from one society to the next, for the obvious reason that societies perish without them. Society must produce an adequate ethic for the same reason it must produce an adequate diet. There are, on the other hand, rules of morality which provide the standards of polite and acceptable behaviour of an age or a culture. Moralities are subject to wide variation with time and among different cultural traditions. Every community has a morality – but it has it as every food has a flavour, not as every diet must contain sufficient calories.

Finding Your Morality

Unlike ethics, which are universal and long-term, any specific morality is applicable only in the short term and to a limited community. It does not matter much for the *existence* of a society – only its flavour. A few people in the world may claim that a different-flavoured culture from their own is

119

unbearable – but probably not very many when the chips are down.

It is not up to me to tell you what your morality should be. It is up to you to find out.

I am not avoiding a responsibility. I would be if I told you specifically what your morality should be. I am doing something more difficult than telling you what you ought to do. I am facing the fact that every mother's son and daughter of us have *in fact* achieved our moralities by our own actions, our own decisions.

There are hundreds of moralities in the modern West. They vary with education and income, with the country or section of the country, with ethnic and racial origin, with religion and the degree to which different individuals cleave to it. There are hundreds of moralities.

And from the standpoint of any one morality, some or even all of the others may be 'wrong'.

How have we in fact found our moralities – those of us who are mature enough to think we have? By discussing them with friends, parents, clergymen, teachers; by overcoming our fears and our curiosities; by understanding our bodies and the rules of our society. And why are we adults afraid for the youngsters? Because we know how precarious and how difficult the job was for us – and will be for them. In our love we want to spare them – and that is sentimental, because we cannot. What we *can* do is to calm our fears, answer their questions, and trust in their good sense.

You, a young person, must look curiously and honestly at the morality of your community. Discuss it with friends, parents, clergymen, teachers – anybody whom you like and respect, and with whom you can talk easily. You are not asking them what you should do, because they cannot tell you. They can tell you what they *hope* you will do, and whether they will *respect* you if you do. But, so long as you remain within the law, and within the rules for breaking rules, they cannot control your behaviour. You do that yourself.

Therefore, the first step is to discover what the rules of your community are. Please notice that I did not ask you to like it or admire it or even to emulate it. But find out, coolly and overtly, what the rules are.

The next question, then, is: What happens to the people who break those rules? Are they ostracized? Beaten? Shamed? Humiliated? Jailed? Executed? How do the rule-breakers react? By leaving? By buckling down? By confessing and going on?

Knowing all these things, then, you decide what you are going to do and what you are not going to do. Be sure, in other words, that you know what your community's morality is, what its demands are, and what your own principles are. Then chart your behaviour. This puts a burden on the individual. It may appear trite, but it is nevertheless true: responsibility is the price of freedom.

Here are just a few of the many questions you must deal with: What will happen to my life if I transgress the rules of the community and am forced to marry? What if pregnancy results and we are not forced to marry? Have I spoiled my chances of ever getting married? What educational opportunities will be curtailed? What social opportunities do I close the door on?

You are not interested in averages – young marriage and young divorce rates, premarital pregnancies, and the like. Your question is: What will happen to you?

Notice that I have not in this book said 'Don't' or 'Wait for marriage'. Most books on this subject advise that. Neither have I said 'Do' or 'Now'. Only charlatans give that advice. I am assuming that young people are mature enough that they can learn what their own morality is. I am assuming that you can live in terms of the ethics of 'do not lead anybody astray and do not allow yourself to be led astray'. I do not predict damage if you decide on premarital intercourse; I do not say damage will not occur, for it sometimes does. I do not predict either marital success or lack of it if you are a virgin at marriage. For some people, in some communities, it is the only moral condition; for others in other communities, it would be intolerable.

Probably at no time in the history of the world has it been so easy for an individual to move from one community to another as in modern America today. Many of us have, by changing our geographical and cultural communities, found or even created *our* community.

But there is a danger. One can be seduced by a new morality just as by a person. Moralities themselves have to be examined for their ethical basis: regard for the rights and autonomy of other people. Is your new morality an unethical morality? That is not an empty question.

People should live with and obey the moral precepts of their communities. The reason is an obvious and selfish one: few people are tough enough to take without great pain the guilt and public opprobrium that comes from flouting the morals and principles of the community. *There's* the rub.

And in a country such as ours, there is little need to. Just as moralities of communities and whole societies change with time and new conditions, so may the moralities of individuals change as they grow older and more experienced. You will probably change your moral position at least once in your life, and perhaps several times. You certainly cannot make up your mind to a morality when you are fifteen and still have it working smoothly when you are forty – finding your morality is a constant aspect of living. But if you change it suddenly or precipitously, you may well be sorry.

What is *not* moral is to refuse to make a commitment to some set of standards. If you repeatedly and constantly allow yourself to drift away from the morality of the community in which you grew up, but have not taken up a new and positive morality of your own, if you make it appear that it is someone else's fault that you are not moral, then what you are doing is unethical. You are kidding yourself. You are insisting that you be seduced so that you can have your cake of imagining yourself a moral person at the same time that you eat your cake by doing things you consider immoral.

'Badness' never comes from the sexual act itself. It comes from dishonesty with yourself and with your partner.

One final point: many societies can and do exist with what seem to us to be weird and strange moralities. In today's Western world, there is a morality gap between generations. I worry about that very little. But I do worry about ethical standards – for no society can continue to exist without them. Ethical behaviour furnishes the basis of social life. Morality gives it tone. Be sure you know the difference.

A Note on Getting Into – and Out of 'Trouble'.

Although most pregnancies – both inside and outside marriage – occur when no contraceptives are used or when they are used ineptly, nevertheless occasionally pregnancies do occur even after precautions are taken. When these pregnancies are non-marital, they are sometimes considered 'tragedies'. Actually, of course, they are no such thing – they are the natural results of natural acts. Pregnancy is proof positive that sexual acts have occurred – it is often the difficulty of living with such explicit proof that makes a problem for a girl and her parents, and even for the boy and his parents. Getting caught is, in such moralities, much 'worse' than the sexual act itself.

Surely, one must accept the entirety of one's sexuality *before* entering into a sexual relationship. The possibility of pregnancy may be made highly improbable with adequate contraception, but it cannot be excluded. Anybody who cannot accept the possible consequences of his action – and pregnancy is a very plain and simple consequence – is not yet able to accept his sexuality *in toto*. It is this fact – this incapacity to accept – which lays the ground for any tragedy.

The problem of dealing with the pregnancy falls on both partners, assuming some stability in the relationship that led to it. The pregnancy is the responsibility of the two people. It is foolish to confuse responsibility with blame. Blaming does not help.

The programme is a simple one: first go to a doctor. If he is not helpful, or if his own morality gets in your way, go to another. Find out if you really are pregnant – 'pseudocyesis' is the name of an illness in which a woman thinks herself pregnant and shows some of the symptoms. If you are not, that takes care of the matter.

123

If you are pregnant, then you have two choices: either you bear the child or you get a medical abortion (*quack abortions really should be ruled out* even from consideration). If you decide to bear the child, then the child must be either placed for adoption or else retained. If the child is retained, the mother can either marry or not marry – her marrying legitimatizes the child, even if her husband did not beget the child.

The question of marriage looms large in the fears of an unwed couple. An outsider can say only that a child's father as well as his mother has a responsibility to him, but that marriage is a state that can be rewarding only when it is undertaken for itself. If the parents-to-be – for so they now are – want to get married on other grounds than the girl's pregnancy, perhaps it is the best solution. If they do not, almost surely it is not a good solution at all.

The polemic against abortion always centres around two points: (1) the taking of life, and (2) permissiveness towards those who get caught. Abortion is a tricky problem because so many legal systems have legislated against it. In the morality that lies behind the law, the question is always, 'When is the human being a human being?' When does the child get a distinctive individuality (read 'soul' if you like) separate from the mother? It is this point on which the debate actually hinges, and one to which a mere medical answer can never be given.

Although ideas about abortion in your community are almost surely 'scarce information', you can discover what the ideas and practices are if you ask the right people – and since the people vary with the community, you have to find them yourself. Ideas about adoption may also be hard to come by. But they can be discovered.

And ultimately, it is of course you alone who have to make up your mind what you are going to do. Don't be pressured one way or the other.

Chapter 14

Marriage

'Marriage' is a social phenomenon as well as a personal commitment. The most important thing about it is that it is the *social* recognition of the union (including sexual union) of a man and a woman. Physically you are no different after marriage than you are before. Socially, however, you are a different 'person'. You are now not only yourself. You are a partner in a legal unit, the married couple, that can hold property before the law; in almost all societies it is the recognized household unit. The partners have legitimate sexual rights in one another (which can be protected legally), and in some societies – including our own – these rights are exclusive. The children borne by the woman (and presumably begotten by the man) are 'legitimate'.

This public recognition of the union of a man and a woman begins with a ceremony – the wedding ceremony turns a liaison into a marriage. The wedding, in our society, is a way of announcing to the world – either quietly, or with considerable social noise, depending on what the individuals want – that a mating is taking place, and that this marriage is receiving the blessing of the community.

Marriage as an End

In the Western world, the ideal situation is that love precedes marriage and that marriage precedes sexual intercourse. Then, after marriage, companionship is supposed to deepen with sexual satisfaction and living together, and children come along in the natural course of events and are welcomed. Marriage begins a new set of even deeper involvements in the experiment in intimacy.

Other societies of the world chain the events of intimacy in somewhat different ways. In traditional China and in parts of Africa, marriages are arranged. In some (but not all) of those societies, love between the married partners is considered highly desirable, but people say that it is impossible to tell whether you have found 'love' before you have been married – perhaps for some years. In those societies your parents and your spouse's parents, or a professional matchmaker, strike an arrangement between two families on some basis that includes a considered judgement about personalities. The young people are then married. If the matchmakers have done their jobs well – and they usually do – the two young people are compatible. The relationship begins with sex, proceeds to children. Living together and having children leads to companionship. Such societies have not made the same one-to-one correlation between love, sex, and marriage as have Westerners, for all that they think the three should go together. Such arranged marriages work well in these societies, because the spouses do not depend so fully on one another for companionship and the necessities of life as spouses do in our society. A man can still depend on his parents; the bride can have the assistance and comfort of her parents and her parents-in-law. This is not 'interfering' as it would be with us.

There is a set of physical purposes or aims which a marriage solves anywhere. It solves the problem of the control as well as the expression of human sexuality, and it does it within a context of maximum dependability, predictability, and (as one wit has added) opportunity. Because marital sexuality is approved by society, it is possible to relax and let love and sex work together. Of course, there are a few people for whom sexuality is made more intense by its very forbidden quality. Sex may, to them, be uninteresting if it is not illicit or irresponsible. Such people miss a lot. To most, sexuality is made more pleasurable by predictable and dependable love, and hence marital sexuality is now and will continue to be usual for most (but not all) mature individuals.

This 'controlled' marital sexuality (which means social control, not curtailed activity on the part of the individual partners with one another) also, obviously, leads to the satisfaction of society's need for reproduction of the species. The family based on marriage is the most secure and most dependable way to recruit the next generation.

There are many other socially important purposes of marriage as well. In the first place, the marriage bond permits the fullness of sexual experience to be brought into balance with the rest of the everyday environment. The couple form a social unit, and in the United States and to a lesser degree in western Europe, the couple solve for one another the primary need for dependable and trusting companionship.

Marriage as a Beginning

Therefore, although marriage solves many problems and ends a search and a period of uncertainty, it is also a beginning. A wedding brings a new social institution – a new family – into existence. And that has its own problems and demands a great adjustment from every person. When you marry, you have indeed solved one set of problems. But you encounter an even bigger set of new problems.

The domestic work of the world can best be done by couples – and their subsequent children – either within a larger extended family, or as individual households. Not only do helpless babies and young children have to be fed, but if the entire labour of feeding and sheltering the population can be divided and organized, then it can all be achieved at much less trouble to each individual. A man and woman form a convenient unit for the division of the labour necessary to do the world's work. Because the woman bears and rears the children, she is confined (for at least some periods of her life) to a smaller orbit of social activity than is a man; almost everywhere the women keep house, doing the cooking and house cleaning and baby-tending, while men wander farther afield and bring in the food. This does not mean that women are not important food producers, for they are in many societies. It does not mean that all women must stay at home. In most hunting societies the products gathered by the women are the stop-gap when men's hunting fails; in many agricultural societies women are the farmers or at the very least carry out some important agricultural tasks. In modern industrial societies, some women are important in industry, education, and government. But in all societies, there is within the household a division of tasks between men and women (and, sometimes, between the generations as well), and that division of tasks makes the man and the woman and their children increasingly dependent on each other.

Perhaps the most important task of the married couple (and perhaps of their parents and siblings as well) is providing a setting to facilitate the maturation of the next generation. When sociologists talk about this, they say that the next generation must be 'socialized' or 'trained'. These facts are, of course, true, but saying it that way leaves out the fact that when the parents are relaxed and secure, children are eager to learn and their socialization is a matter of division of responsibility between parents and children.

And that is what marriage is about: the predictable, approved, and loving expression of sexuality, producing the next generation, providing companionship and a trustworthy social unit, getting the world's work done and its people fed and housed, educating the children as they mature physically and psychically, and providing them with a secure and predictable world.

The Plagues of Marriage

There are a number of what might be called diseases of marriage – 'false' uses to which marriage can be put. These diseases are sometimes difficult to diagnose until infection is far advanced. First of all, there is the illusion called 'happiness'. Marriage is not about happiness. Marriages are sometimes happy – but if they are, it is because both parties to the marriage carry out their jobs with good will and at least a modicum of effectiveness and enjoyment. That leads to contentment, dependability and to greater love, from all of which much happiness can be garnered. Marriage is about the job of rearing children with full attention, and with love, so that the children grow into effective mature individuals – that also makes great happiness. It is about the companionship that is felt and not feigned, when both partners are completely open and uninhibited in their sexuality, and when the division of tasks is done adequately and cheerfully. In such a situation, it takes a real grouch not to be happy. But, of course, no real grouch would ever find himself in that position.

There is another disease of marriage that is even more difficult to detect in its early stages, and hence difficult to prevent. That occurs when two people come to depend on one another not because it makes life easier and richer and more pleasant, but because they would perish – physically or at least psychically – without one another. This is a neurotic dependence.

All successfully married persons should and do depend on one another. But that does not mean that (on most occasions – certainly on routine occasions) they are not capable of coping independently of one another. A woman who does not know how to behave without her husband, and who is afraid of new experiences, may come to have a neurotic dependence on him; similarly a man who is afraid of other women and uses his wife as a shield against them or who, for some deep-seated reason, finds it necessary constantly to do things for her so that she will in turn 'mother' him also has a neurotic dependence. Let it be repeated – for married people to depend on one another is normal and good; but for them to use that dependence to keep from being fully dependable themselves, in all aspects of life, is a disease of marriage and one of the most difficult to 'cure'.

The best cure for neurotic dependence is to avoid it by marrying someone who will not reciprocate it. However, that is very difficult, and for two reasons: first, because, like cancer, it may grow from what appear to be normal processes; and second, because it usually takes two of a kind to bring it off – and in such a condition, you are the last to know. If anybody tries to tell you before marriage that you have made a poor choice, try to listen.

Try to evaluate what that person's point is in telling you. It may be a real interest in you and your future (and, unfortunately, it may not be). But try to listen – and do not get defensive or stubborn. And, also, try to listen to yourself: most of the divorced people I have interviewed, who had escaped from being locked into these unfortunate marriages, claim that they knew before marriage about the possibility of difficulties, but chose to overlook it because being married was so important to them.

One of the most deadly of all the plagues of marriage is jealousy – the idea seems to crop up that something in the marriage ceremony is supposed to make everybody except the spouse unattractive. Obviously, nothing could be further from the truth. What we have to do is to make a distinction between what we feel and what we do – and remember that it is possible to feel something without doing anything – and hence without being guilty of any wrong. Wrong may result from acts or their omission but not from mere feelings (unless, of course, they lead to 'wrong acts'). Petty jealousy on the part of a woman because her husband finds other women attractive is no more than a vulgar display of self-doubt. If he actually does find other people attractive, she may be glad that he finds her more so – or at least that he did once and probably will again. If a man is jealous of every other man his wife smiles at, he will soon, necessarily, have her turned into an unsmiling and not very attractive woman, or a woman no longer attracted to him.

Jealousy after marriage can often be predicted before marriage. The first 'symptom' is that the couple are, during their courtship, primarily intent on escaping from other people. I do not mean, obviously, that it isn't right and normal to want to be alone when you are courting. I mean, rather, that for such a couple the chief goal in courting is to shut out all the rest of the world for good. This syndrome usually begins with hostility to parents and teachers. After escape from the parents, the hostility is directed to the peers. And if a marriage takes place that actually allows escape from the peers, then the hostility is always directed toward the spouse.

One of the most serious diseases of marriage to be found

today is peculiar to very young couples. When very young people marry, they have a job to do that is additional to the ordinary jobs of marriage and the ordinary adventures in intimacy: they must grow and develop socially and psychically in tune with one another. That may be true of all marriages, but it is particularly true of young marriages, because young people cannot yet have found their social selves completely. Young people sometimes marry for what seem to be good reasons, but find later that they have used this road as a short cut to a sort of forged adulthood.

Young Americans, for example, do not become adult all at once, at some grand initiation. They begin paying adult prices at movies when they are twelve. They can get a driver's licence when they are sixteen. If they are males, they can be drafted at eighteen. They can get married without permission when they are sixteen or eighteen – in some states, as low as thirteen for girls. They can buy alcohol when they are twenty-one (except in New York, where they need be only eighteen); and they can vote when they are twenty-one. Americans – and Europeans share this experience – are not promoted into adulthood, but rather they are slowly escalated into it. Somewhere along the line they also must finish their education and become economically independent.

Indeed, social maturity does not occur today until about twenty-four or twenty-five years of age – it is, in fact, a constant and lifelong process – because there is so much education to be got, and so much culture to master. Sometimes boys and girls think they can hasten this process by getting married. They reason that since the mark of a mature person is marriage, they will get married and automatically become mature.

Nobody doubts that adolescents can fall deeply and sincerely in love. But most adults *do* doubt that love is the *only* requirement for marriage. Most married adolescents grow up to this extent – they learn to agree with the adults on *that* point.

Selecting a Mate

People tend to select partners who meet particular needs of their own. This is true, even when you do not like a particular characteristic in yourself or in the partner. Nevertheless, at one level these needs must be met. Therefore, in every case the characteristics and qualities of the person whom you consciously choose to marry are accompanied with a set of qualities and characteristics that you have unconsciously selected.

Therefore, in our society, *you* made the selection. And you do it with your whole personality, not just the conscious part. Remember that when the marriage occurs, there is more to it than you know about. And whatever that unconscious foundation may be, it will become more so and more so.

Marriage in the Western world is based on love. But it is not based on love alone. It is based on the entire range of needs and drives of the individuals. It must include as an important element two people's capacities to lead non-dependent adult lives, a capacity to make at least one living, and sufficient mental and social experience and knowledge on the part of both spouses that they can be good parents.

If you are a normally outgoing person who is sure of himself and esteems his own capabilities and goals and ambitions, and if you listen to the comments and suggestions of those around you, you will make a good marriage. If you are too hostile, instead of just normally aggressive, if you do not esteem yourself, and if you are searching for a 'way out', you probably will not.

Marriage is a last resort – if you can possibly solve your problems any other way, don't get married.

Marriages can lead to great happiness, but that is not the purpose of marriage – its purpose is to regulate (which, for individuals, means to enhance) sexual conduct, to provide the domestic necessities of a household, to create a family by begetting the next generation and providing an atmosphere in which the capacity to love and the desire for training and education lead into responsible adulthood. A good marriage demands constant work – and it is one of the few things that is its own reward.

But when you do it, remember this one other thing: you are not getting rid of your problems. They will come with you. And you are taking on a whole new set of obligations that have problems of their own.

Chapter 15

The Family

It is man's fate to be born into a family. It is every individual's particular fate to be born into a particular family.

The Biological Basis of the Human Family

The family is as much a part of man's biological nature as is his upright stature, his capacity to walk on two legs, the fine co-ordination of eye and hand, and the specialization in brain that makes symbolic thought and language possible.

The biological naturalness of the family derives from two sources: first, human beings, like other mammals, suckle and teach their young. This gives rise to a basic and profound mother-child relationship. Second, sexual desire and activity are not limited to any specific season, but are always present, which gives rise to more or less permanent mating. Since the mother-child relationship is so intimate a one, the sexual relationship is also experienced as an intimate one; the mates prize stability over time in this most intimate of relationships, and have invented marriage.

The mature female feels a biological urge towards her children as well as a sexual attraction towards the male. The male feels a sexual attraction for the female and comes to accept her children and to play an important role in their lives as well as in hers. Paternal instinct is not a biological one, as the maternal instinct is, but something very like it is learned in all human societies.

Two biological drives thus form the underpinning of the human family: continual sexuality and the long period of helplessness and learning in the young. The form of the family changes from one human society to another, but we know today that it changes within very narrow limits: that the maternal instinct and the sex drive lie at its basis; that cultural values and habits are taken in by the child in his relationship with his mother, and that in this process he is himself turned into a family creature. The family will continue to exist among human beings – we are not evolving away from it, no matter how many moralizers mistakenly decry the imminent demise of family life, assuming that its change is its collapse.

The Social Foundations of the Human Family

Every child, because he is a mammal and specifically a human being, is born into a going concern – his family is there before he enters it. The biology of his heredity and – even more importantly – the manner of his upbringing in that family determine the kind of person that he is. In most cases, a person leaves a family behind at death. He thereby also leaves a going concern.

Any family, then, is an entity greater than its individual members, at the same time that (at any given moment) it is made up of the relationships among its members. Americans emphasize the individual and the importance of the family to the individual. People of some other cultures – India, for example, or traditional China – emphasize the importance of the family and the individual loyalty to the family. Yet, these are different institutionalized attitudes to what is fundamentally the same thing.

Not only is a child born into a family living in a single household and containing the mother and father and brothers and sisters. He is also born into a more extended family – a network of aunts, uncles, cousins, grandparents that will later also contain his sons and daughters, nephews and nieces. In some societies many or all of these people may live together and be a major part of every individual's learning about living. In America these more distant kinsmen may be visited only on special occasions. There are many kinds of families, but everybody has one, even though a few people repudiate their families.

Love, Sex and Being Human

What is true is that every culture and every society must spend a certain amount of time worrying about and working at the quality of its family life. Americans typically do this worrying by prophesying the ruin or the end of the family; these prophecies then allow them to buckle down to work. The expectations in family life in America are very high – higher perhaps than they have ever been before. The nostalgic 'myth' of the old-fashioned family that 'stayed together' is largely just that – a myth. The myth is also, like the worrying and the dire predictions, a necessary means by which we can hold the standards of perfection up to ourselves.

Because of our long childhoods, the amount we have to learn, and because we belong to a species to which the family is a natural form, our social selves are almost as predetermined in this way as our body chemistry is given by our cells. Yet, you can change vast reaches of your social self by education and by retraining yourself to new ideas and values. Whole societies and cultures change and develop. For all that, a person's basic personality is still influenced by his earliest family experiences, no matter what he does later. The family experience is a framework, like the biological framework, within which the human individual and the human species must win its victories and take its rewards.

The Family Household

Every society creates households based on family groups. There are many different forms of household groups in different societies depending on the rules of that society about which kinsmen any person lives with. But households everywhere are composed of a limited number of the available kinsmen, and they are always the most important groups in shaping the social self of every individual. You share intimate experiences with the members of your household – and with the other people in your society who were brought up in similar households.

The family, in the household, sorts people out and gives them instruction in their roles, according to age, sex, and sort – the

136

latter in the sense of class and the sense of family specialties or peculiarities.

The Western family today is unusual in the history of the world because its household contains such a small segment of the total family group. In the most prized of the many ways of living, only a couple and their children live together. That fact means that a child grows up in constant and very intense touch with his parents and his brothers and sisters – and usually not with anyone else. Such a family has real rewards – especially for the parents. Its rewards for children are less entrancing, because there is nobody to escape to if mother is ill or if father is grouchy or if big brother takes all the toys. There is no one to teach basic attitudes and skills when the parents lack them or neglect the job. Schools can provide some of the necessary training, but not all of it. The nuclear family household, as it is called, undoubtedly curtails the experience of children, and creates the necessity for children to depend more fully and earlier on outside contacts, and then to rebel more obviously and perhaps more violently at the time of adolescence.

Adolescent Rebellion

However, this form of household also achieves something else, which most of us (at least) all regard as good. It means that in the process of growing up, the child can become an equal with his parents. He can become their colleague. In no society with an extended family household is this particular form of individual autonomy either required or possible. In those societies the child remains dependent no matter what his age, so long as the father and other older kinsmen are alive or at least until they retire.

Middle-class people of Europe and America say that young people must be ready for a family when they marry. That does not mean merely that they are physically developed sufficiently to beget and bear children. It does not even mean merely that they are economically able to maintain a household. It means also that the social and personal revolution of adolescence has been satisfactorily achieved: that one has in fact become an autonomous individual, preferably one who has returned to his parents and is on an equal footing with them. Children must learn to rebel against their parents without leaving them (either figuratively or literally – I do not mean that they should not get an apartment of their own, but rather that they should for their own good not cut themselves off completely); they must also learn to do it without hating their parents.

Just as important, parents must learn to let their children rebel – and that means to be a good and worthy adversary to them so that they can come back as equals. This is a difficult point in parenthood – if a child is encouraged to rebel, he is unable to do it. If a child is held down too tightly by whatever means, he is unable to do it. A parent must call upon his own security and capacity to love in this case as much as he ever did earlier in his child's life.

This particular adolescent revolt, which every American (and, perhaps to a lesser degree, every European) must go through, is difficult for the adolescent as well. It is what the psychoanalyst Erik Erikson has called the search for identity. When a young person has found out who he is, he can then come back to his parents as their equal – not their boss or their 'child', but as an adult son or daughter who has through the skill and love of his parents become skilful and loving and has established his own self-esteem independent now of the parental regard for him. This is what Americans call 'growing up'.

This kind of growing up is necessary if one is to found a family and a household of one's own that is fully rewarding and fully efficient.

No fully successful new family or household can be formed by people who have not completed this adolescent revolt. Perhaps (but I am not convinced) it is not impossible to lay the groundwork after marriage; certainly it is very much more difficult. I do not mean, of course, that it is absolutely necessary for the parents to approve one's choice of mate – but if the revolt and return are successfully completed, they usually do. I repeat: it is sometimes the fault of the parent that the adolescent rebellion cannot be successfully achieved and the new *entente* cordially and profitably made. Yet, it is nevertheless the responsibility of the child. No child should blame a parent for the difficulty until he has exhausted all other explanations.

Many of the difficulties in American families come in the next generation, when this process of becoming a colleague of the parent is not achieved. Many young people who have not in fact achieved this process are capable of love. And many can treat the first few years of their marriage much like a love affair. But, especially with the birth of children, the difficulty re-emerges. You are now the parent instead of the child – but the unresolved relationship is the same and has come home to roost. You cannot be a satisfactory parent until you have been through the process of being a satisfactory child – best with your own parents, but it is possible to do it vicariously. Merely turning your back on your parents is not enough.

The Functions and Purposes of Families

The family in Europe and America, thus, is a small, nuclear family. Never has so much depended on so few. It is sometimes said – even by social scientists who should know better – that the family is coming to have less and less responsibility or purpose as schools and other special organizations take over the responsibilities that were formerly in the realm of the family. An expert should not accept such ideas merely because they are found among the people in his samples – when he picks up a message, he ought to listen for the cry for help as well as the datum he had in mind.

The real question is more subtle: in a society in which so many special techniques are taught by non-family members, how does the family teach the basic concepts of ethics, morality, and motivation? In a primitive society, a boy has to be taught to shoot a bow and arrow, and must grow up knowing the requirements for his niche in society. In our middle class family, a boy has to be taught to be the kind of person who can go to university, and who can get and hold a responsible job – he must be given the capacity to discover and make his niche in society. There is no doubt in my mind about which is more difficult and which requires a greater devotion to family life: it is the latter. The problem is simple to state but difficult to deal with: when children learn so few basic techniques from their parents, what are the parents to use as a matrix for teaching the ethics and the motivations toward hard work? Example, of course – but it is sometimes not enough.

One of the most important things that we learn in families is how to be parents. Children are taught the parental roles at the same time they are taught the child roles. And in that fact lies the real toughness of the human family. The family is the smallest group that can do *everything* (except, of course, provide a spouse). It is what the scientists would call 'elegant' – the smallest number of people, organized for maximum rewards and maximum effectiveness. It seems doubtful if the number of people can be reduced and the family retain either the effectiveness or the rewards.

The family is, as we can see, not only the fate of every individual, it is the basic social institution. It is the natural form of human social grouping because it allows conservation of energy and maximization of stability.

Family Disruption

Therefore, in talking and learning about the morality of sex, it is impossible for human beings not to concentrate on the idea of the family. It is also impossible, however, for them not to consider two related ideas: (1) what happens when family life goes wrong, and (2) sex outside the family and what the moralities of the world permit.

There is no denying that sometimes things go wrong in families. In every marriage, in every family, there are times when one thinks one is giving more than one is getting (it may be true for long periods of time), and there are times when tedium sets in. Occasionally people want to break out of their families. Sometimes some of them do so – children leave home in anger; adultery occurs; marriages break up.

All societies limit extramarital sex more or less stringently. Some demand that people live up to these limitations; others do not. Our own society is in the majority in that it does not have any institutionalized and favoured form of extramarital sexual activity (a few societies do have, usually but not always in connexion with ceremonies or specific periods of license). In fact, extramarital sex is both condemned and, to some degree, practised in our society.

If one partner does commit adultery the world of the other need not collapse. Talk about it – preferably with the offending spouse. But it should be remembered that very few people indeed commit adultery if their marriages are completely satisfactory, and it almost always takes two people to make an unsatisfactory marriage. No – not always; but usually. Adultery is not the automatic end of a marriage – but it is a ground for divorce and is often used as a means of kidding one's self.

I hope it is obvious that I am not condoning adultery. I hope it is equally obvious that we should – in the middle class at least – treat repeated and constant adultery as a symptom of serious marital difficulty. And still equally obvious that every married person must come to realize that the spouse's body remains the property of the spouse. The one-flesh metaphor can be carried too far. Marriage is a relationship; it is only socially and metaphorically a 'union'. Like all relationships, it is coloured by what people think and feel, and the emotions that they experience. But it *is* what people do.

Divorce

Sometimes spouses divorce one another. Divorce is not in itself evil by any except particular religious definitions, which make marriage a sacrament as well as a fundamental social relationship. Divorce is socially and individually harmful (which means something quite different) only if the tasks that are ordinarily performed by the family are not carried out by somebody else in cases of divorce.

Nobody questions that the best arrangement – because it is

both moral and economical – is for families to proceed to do their jobs and end up with a sense of accomplishment and perhaps also of happiness.

But sometimes people do not or cannot live in specific family situations. Living in constant strife is debilitating. Although divorce should not be 'easy' (whatever that means) we should not be afraid of it. We may regret it – we cannot help regretting it. But we need not fear it. We should not (and will not) promote it or be in favour of it. That does not mean that we should turn our backs on recognizing it and its problems or make scapegoats of the people who become involved in it. When people divorce, they should be prepared to carry out their responsibilities as best they can. If it is difficult to carry out those responsibilities in marriage, it is even more difficult to carry them out in a divorce. But nevertheless divorces do occur, and it does no good at all to moan about them, and it may be worse than no good to try to 'save' marriages that are truly destructive to the people (including the children) involved in them.

It is sometimes said that it is the children who suffer at the time of divorce. That is often true. But that does not mean that we should merely feel sorry for those children, or even that we should make it necessary for their parents to stay together if they cannot possibly live amicably with one another. It means, rather, that we have a job to do in finding ways in which such children can be given the training and the security that they would have got in a two-parent home.

The new art of marriage counselling needs to be improved and expanded – as marriage counsellors and family therapists are the first to agree. But it also needs a more informed public on which to work: a public that realizes that marital difficulties, except in the most disrupted of cases, are difficulties in communications and in goals and motivations which can be talked out and made overt. The public also needs to know that some marriages actually have proceeded to the point that individual psychic damage is unavoidable if they continue. We have to think and care about all the vast morality of marriage, not just an unthinking 'Marriages must be saved'. Lives and sanities must be saved. That is usually most easily and most rewardingly done by renegotiating marriages – but not always.

The even greater demand is for us to put our minds to the social innovation necessary to keep the children of divorce (and the divorced partners themselves) from suffering. If keeping their parents together fails – or never had a chance of succeeding – then the children must still be given the benefits that every human being needs to be human, and hence deserves: the training to master his culture and the security to grow into a self-esteemed individual.

The family, in short, is the basic molecule of any human society. The forms of the family will continue to vary and perhaps to change. The demands on families may change – probably to increase and become more abstract as specialist functions are taken over by specialist institutions. African societies may continue to practise polygamy. Chinese societies may continue to respect the extended family (in spite of communism and industrialization). American society may continue to live in fragmented nuclear family households which require what some Europeans call domestic overcapitalization and which psychiatrists agree demands the intensification of the adolescent rebellion. But all societies that endure will have a family.

Once and for all, sexuality lies at the basis of family life. And, of precisely equal importance, family life lies at the basis of sexuality. The family is the human response to sexuality and to the many responsibilities, feelings, and pleasures that it implies. The two are linked – they are, in fact, part of the same thing (though each extends outside the other). It is possible, once one is adult, to live without a family; a few people choose to do so. Given the services that are commercially available in the modern world, it is possible and sometimes even rewarding. But for most people, the family is the core of all life – it is what human life is about.

Chapter 16

Finding Your Own Morality

Only a couple of generations ago, people were frightened into a moral posture instead of educated about an ethical way of living.

We should all be grateful that the age of mystification is gone. Sex is not charged with mystery or danger – it is the mystification itself which is the mystery.

The old attitudes of fear were maintained by the threat of unwanted pregnancy or of venereal disease. Today we know about effective methods of contraception. No method is 100 per cent effective, but properly used, both hormone pills and intra-uterine devices approach it.

Similarly, venereal disease is not the scourge it once was. True – the rate of venereal disease has been going up since the late 1950s, when it was almost wiped out, and the infection rate is highest among middle class teenagers. But today we know how to cure most venereal disease – though a few strains are resistant to antibiotics. VD today is largely a result of careless and unethical standards. Obviously, the ethical position is that if you find yourself infected, you go to a doctor and do not have any further sexual relations until the disease has been cured.

This new enlightenment – built firmly on the pill and the intra-uterine device and on antibiotics – has allowed us to see the real problem for the first time in history. Today, the only basis for morality is knowledge and ethical conviction - based on regard for others. Just as obviously, real morality was *always* based on such a foundation. The difference today is that we cannot escape moral decisions simply by deciding (instead) to avoid illegitimacy, forced marriage, or syphilis.

The Search for Morality

There is an old saying in the English-speaking countries: a stiff penis has no conscience. Every such saying has a 'moral' – a lesson that is to be heeded (and the fact that the word for it is a 'moral' should not be overlooked). The moral to this old saying is: the ethical and moral dimensions of your sexual behaviour should be determined and dealt with *before* you enter into a sexual relationship, marital or non-marital, not afterwards.

The search for your sexual morality – whoever 'you' may be – involves three sets of facts: (1) the facts of biology, including contraception, (2) the facts of your community traditions and your place in the community, including both the ideal rules and the rules for compromising them, and (3) some mature consideration of your own goals and principles.

Your own morality is the particular adjustment of these three forces that makes it possible for you to live with maximum self-esteem (the source, after all, of love and lovableness, of respect and respectability).

Your own search for facts. The basic facts of the biology of sex and reproduction have been given earlier. If you want more information, a list of some books will be found in the appendix.

The ideal demands of your community morality you already know. By talking to friends, teachers, parents, clergymen, you can discover (if they are honest) what the rules for breaking the rules are. If they are not honest with you, then it is one of the moral principles of your community to be dishonest in some matters (and you can perhaps find a way to set about changing that).

It should be recognized, however, that some adults find great difficulty in discussing sex with their children. If you are such a parent, the honest statement is 'I have great trouble in talking about this – please get the facts from a doctor.' Then help your child to find the right doctor. If you are a doctor who feels inadequate or uncomfortable about this subject, then refer the child (or adult) to another doctor who can and will do it well.

If you are a clergyman who finds discussion of these topics difficult or upsetting, look into the many classes that are being held for clergymen in universities and in seminaries on counselling about these very topics.

It is not dishonest or humiliating to say that you find discussing these matters difficult. It *is* dishonest of you and humiliating for the young person if you fob him off with mystification or embarrassed inanities.

Your Own Goals and Principles

Harold Laski wrote somewhere that freedom is release from whatever bonds are currently most pressing and confining. We might add that bliss appears as the whole set of good things that you do not currently have. The most frequent difficulty in establishing your own goals is that you get them confused with freedom and bliss.

For many young people, the most pressing problem is being adolescent. Their most keenly felt lacks are lack of love and esteem, and lack of approved sex. The danger is that they will combine these two and decide that freedom from adolescence can best be attained by sexual bliss. Indeed, I think that the current trend towards younger marriages is triggered in part by this very confusion: some young people try to marry themselves out of adolescence into bliss. It is a mark of maturity that you know that freedom is the opportunity to recognize and choose your own limitations, and that bliss is a fantasy designed to hide both intellectual and emotional understanding of your current situation.

Some Questions to Ask Yourself. A list of topics about which you have to be clear is to be found in Table 3. At any time in your adult life, you should have a pretty clear idea about where you stand on all of these points: about what your goals are, and how you would like to handle them, and about the rules for compromise.

In working out these questions and topics, it came as something

Table 3. The Dimensions of Sexual Morality

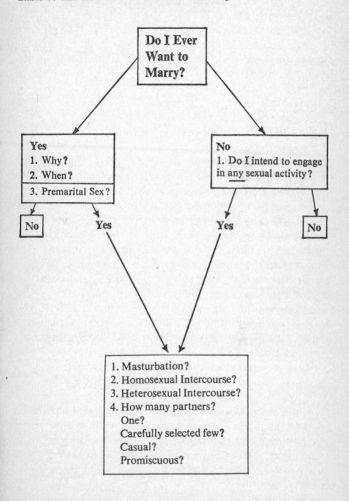

of a surprise to me to find that the question of marriage is indeed the central question: DO I EVER WANT TO GET MARRIED, AT ALL, TO ANYBODY? It is central for a simple but powerful reason: the answer to this question determines whether you look on your sexual acts as premarital or as nonmarital.

There are, in modern America and probably in every other society, two moral universes – that of the married and that of the unmarried. It is the mark of an advanced civilization that we can even ask the question: do I want to get married – ever?

Being Single. There are two sets of considerations about singleness: one has to do with the rewards and the price of mobility and non-attachment; the other has to do with the way in which you consider personal intimacy. What are you going to do about housing arrangements and the kind of exchange of services that being married implies? What are you going to do about companionship? What are you going to do about sex?

In a recent long report on the subject, *Time* magazine went into the whole subject of the 'swinging singles' who have become a fashionable (and consumption-oriented) segment of the American population. What *Time* reporters found is that some single people – but by no means the majority – have a smashing time during the years of their singleness and are single because they want to be. A greater number are single, after twenty-five or so, in spite of the fact that they do not want to be. With fairly relaxed sexual standards and a fairly high income, many have a good time, by their own lights. Yet, many of them intend to marry; some of those who do not, discover – sometimes to their own amazement – that by the time they are in their late twenties they are tired and a little bored, and that the world looks different.

However, it is possible to be single in our culture today, either for long periods of time or permanently. It is not an unrewarding life, and it is certainly not a depressed one. The necessary domestic services can be bought on the open market – apartments with cleaning service, frozen foods (or gourmet cooking parties), and good laundries are available in all cities, and in many small towns. Companionship is not hard to come by, if you have any talent at all for finding companions. Sex is an issue that you can decide for yourself, so long as you stay within the law and the bounds of ethics and decorum. Therefore, aside from parenthood itself, you *may* consider that you are not giving up anything by staying single (but you may also discover that you are).

Being Married. Marriage solves some of the problems of being single – it provides a ready-made set of mutual services and householding chores; it provides an answer to the need for intimacy. It provides built-in companionship. It offers the promise of a rewarding sexual relationship without a perennial quest.

Marriage, however, is not bliss or happiness. It involves compromise – you must restructure your social universe to overlap with somebody else's. It can provide a setting in which sex is given maximum security and maximal expression; it can provide a setting in which companionship is maximal. It can provide a legitimate place to be a parent.

Do not expect that you will not change your mind about the question of marriage. You may. If you do, know why.

The rest of the questions in Table 3 are all dependent on the answer to the question of marriage. The sexual acts are the same, whether you are married or not, whether you intend to marry or not. But your attitude towards them cannot possibly be the same.

There are many decent ways to arrange your life in today's world. If you go through the questions on the chart, and are comfortable with what you arrive at – and if it is ethical, as we have talked about ethics in this book – then I am not going to worry about you, whatever you do. If you are uncomfortable or unethical, then somewhere you have done something wrong – wrong for you, and perhaps wrong for society. These questions may not be the right ones for you – no set of questions can be right for everybody. But if some of them are not right, then obviously *you must improve the questions.*

In itself neither sexual activity nor continence is physically harmful. Therefore, morality is a social and cultural matter. Social and cultural matters are as much based on facts as are biological matters. The difference is one of choice. As a biological creature, most of the choices have been made for you. As a social creature, you can make some of your own. The limitations are your biological nature and the demands of your community. The goal is to live with yourself cheerfully and comfortably, whatever that means, within the limitations provided. You have to know the cost of alternatives.

A lot of your elders are going to say that I am taking all the romance out of sex. Your response may well be: 'Great!' By secure knowledge and sensible choices we are taking the fear and mystery out of it. If mystery and romance are the same thing, then romance has got to go. However, if romance means complete abandonment in complete emotional awareness and responsibility – and for the new generation it seems to me that it does – then the world has never been so magnificently romantic as it is today.

The *theme* of this book is that knowledge is necessary for success or pleasure.

The *moral* of this book is that while sex is one of the great pleasures of mankind, you cannot either give or receive the greatest pleasure if you are ignorant about what you are doing, or if you act unethically by 'making things worse' for yourself or for somebody else. Ignorance and bad ethics lead to preoccupation – either with your own morality, or with worry about possible unwanted outcomes for yourself or others. Preoccupation may arise from many sources, but with young people it most often arises from concern about whether what they are doing is 'right', whether they will be 'caught', what punishments may be inflicted, and what the psychic and social costs of this moment of excitement – perhaps of ecstasy – may be. Knowledge and ethics enhance sexual enjoyment by taking away the preoccupation.

People who do not find a good sexual partner miss a lot. The search is a vitally important one in the lives of young people – and some older people too. It is doubtful whether trial and error in bed is the best method of finding a good sexual partner – for the simple reason that genital sex is not the whole of sexuality, let alone of the partnership. It is one role in a complex relationship, which also contains the roles of the companion, the friend, the roommate, and, ultimately perhaps, the co-parent.

There is no better way to end this book than with some lines of Whitman's hymn to sex, to love, to morality, and to humanity:

Through you I drain the pent-up rivers of myself,
In you I wrap a thousand onward years,
On you I graft the grafts of the best-loved of me and America,
The drops I distil upon you shall grow fierce and athletic girls, new artists, musicians, and singers,
The babes I beget upon you are to beget babes in their turn,
I shall demand perfect men and women out of my love-spendings, I shall expect them to interpenetrate with others, as I and you interpenetrate now,
I shall count on the fruits of the gushing showers of them, as I count on the fruits of the gushing showers I give now,
I shall look for loving crops from the birth, life, death, immortality, I plant so lovingly now.

Appendix: Further Reading

1. Anatomy of Sexual Organs:

Ernest Gardner, Donald J. Gray, and Ronan O'Rahilly, *Anatomy: A Regional Study of Human Structure*, 2nd edition. W. B. Saunders, 1963.

Russell T. Woodburne, *Essentials of Human Anatomy*, 3rd edition Oxford University Press, 1965.

Sigmund Grollman, *The Human Body: Its Structure and Physiology*, Collier-Macmillan Company, 1964.

2. Physiology of Sex:

William H. Masters, M.D., and Virginia E. Johnson, *Human Sexual Response*, Churchill, 1966.

Mary Jane Sherfey, M.D., 'The Evolution and Nature of Female Sexuality in Relation to Psychoanalytic Theory.' *Journal of the American Psychoanalytic Association*, Vol. 14, No. 1, January 1966.

3. Heredity, Genetics, and Evolution:

George and Muriel Beadle, *The Language of Life*, Victor Gollancz, 1966.

Bernard G. Campbell, *Human Evolution, An Introduction to Man's Adaptation*, Heinemann Educational, 1967.

4. Life Before Birth:

Geraldine Lux Flanagan, *The First Nine Months of Life*, Heinemann Medical, 1963.

George W. Corner, *Ourselves Unborn, an Embryologist's Essay on Man*, Yale University Press, New Haven, 1944.

William F. Windle, *Physiology of the Fetus*, W. B. Saunders Company, Philadelphia, 1940.

Appendix: Further Reading

5. Moralities:

Bronislaw Malinowski, *The Sexual Life of Savages in North-Western Melanesia.* Originally printed in 1929; Routledge & Kegan Paul.

I. Schapera, *Married Life in an African Tribe,* Faber & Faber, 1966.

Alastair Heron, ed., *Toward a Quaker View of Sex: An Essay by a Group of Friends*, Friends Home Service, 1963.

6. Families:

Virginia Satir, *Conjoint Family Therapy*, Science and Behavior Books, Inc., Palo Alto, 1964.

William J. Goode, *The Family*, Prentice-Hall, 1964.

More About Penguins and Pelicans

Penguinews, which appears every month, contains details of all the new books issued by Penguins as they are published. From time to time it is supplemented by *Penguins in Print*, which is a complete list of all books published by Penguins which are in print. (There are well over three thousand of these.)

A specimen copy of *Penguinews* will be sent to you free on request, and you can become a subscriber for the price of the postage – 4s. for a year's issues (including the complete lists). Just write to Dept EP, Penguin Books Ltd, Harmondsworth, Middlesex, enclosing a cheque or postal order, and your name will be added to the mailing list. Some other Pelicans are described on the following pages.

Note: *Penguinews* and *Penguins in Print* are not available in the U.S.A. or Canada

Boys and Sex

Wardell B. Pomeroy

In this new Pelican, Dr Pomeroy, co-author of the two
Kinsey reports, advises and informs adolescent boys, from
an impartial and unbiased standpoint, on their natural
sex-drives.

Dealing in a clear and honest manner with all aspects of
sexual development, from masturbation and homosexuality
to petting and intercourse, and with an enlightening
'question and answer' section, this book will guide boys
towards a guilt-free understanding of the emotions and
reactions which they will experience throughout puberty.

At no time does Dr Pomeroy pose as the stern moralist:
his aim is to overcome the guilt and anxiety which he feels
are the enemies of a healthy sex life, and, as he states, to
'convey to children a sense of self-respect, responsibility,
openness and the pleasurableness of sex.'

Not for sale in the U.S.A. or Canada

The Sexual Behaviour of Young People

Michael Schofield

This report sets out to supply facts in an area in which sensation has tended to flourish. Michael Schofield's findings are based on the results of some 2,000 interviews held in England with young people between the ages of thirteen and nineteen.

The first fact to emerge is that sexual promiscuity, though it certainly exists, is not a prominent feature of teenage behaviour. Consequently the risk of venereal disease among the young is not high: infections, it is true, have increased lately, but less in this age-group than in others. Illegitimacy, according to this report, presents a graver problem: of every three girls who have premarital sexual intercourse, one can expect to become pregnant.

Scare reports about immorality and disease have raised a cry for improved sex education. Statistics given in this book certainly suggest that the majority of adolescents still receive little or no guidance from parents or teachers. The facts of contraception and venereal disease are almost outside their ken.

Michael Schofield's meticulous and balanced survey provides the kind of evidence (and the stimulus) needed for framing a sound plan of education and advice about sex for the young.

Not for sale in the U.S.A.

Sexual Deviation

Anthony Storr

This book is a brief account of the common types of sexual behaviour which are generally considered perverse or deviant, together with explanations of their origins.

Sado-masochism, fetishism, and other types of sexual deviation are often assumed by the public to be the result either of satiety or else of inordinate desire. It is not generally understood that the unhappy compulsions which plague the deviant person are evidence of an inability to achieve normal sexual relationships, and that such people deserve compassion rather than condemnation.

In this new Pelican, Anthony Storr, the author of *The Integrity of the Personality*, shows how sexual deviations can result from inner feelings of sexual guilt and inferiority which have persisted from childhood. This is within everybody's understanding. It may seem a far cry from the lover's pinch to the whip of the sado-masochist, but embryonic forms of even the most bizarre deviations can be shown to exist in all of us.

Everyone who is interested in sex – and which of us is not? – will be interested in this authoritative account, not only because it explains the sexual feelings of others, but also because it illumines some of their own.

Also available
Integrity of the Personality

Sex in Society

Alex Comfort

Is the proper end of sex procreation or play – or are both
improper? Should every effort be made to do away with the
physical and legal handicaps of venereal disease and
illegitimacy – or are they valuable moral safeguards? Is the
fig-leaf and four-letter-word fixation which distinguishes
much censorship the result of altruism – or of fear?
Does the middle-class background of many social workers
help them to understand other sexual codes? For how
long and with what effect on health is sexual abstinence
possible? Is chastity any more a virtue than malnutrition?

One more question: do people think rationally about sex?
It is Dr Comfort's contention in this book that most of
them do not. 'The main educative task', he writes, 'is one
of emotional deflation, the letting in of sense and study to
replace stereotyped responses.' This task he performs
with clarity, humanity, and – most mercifully – wit.

'It is packed with information, it is cogently and concisely
argued, and many of its sentences stay in the memory
because of the skill with which they are expressed' –
Anthony Storr in the *Sunday Times*

Not for sale in the U.S.A.